WHO CARES?

WHO CARES?

The Changing Health Care System

Judy Lumby
RN, PhD, MHPEd, BA, FCN (NSW), FRCNA

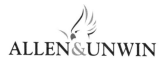

ALLEN&UNWIN

Allen & Unwin
83 Alexander Street
Crows Nest NSW 2065
Australia
Phone: (61 2) 8425 0100
Fax: (61 2) 9906 2218
Email: info@allenandunwin.com
Web: www.allenandunwin.com

National Library of Australia
Cataloguing-in-Publication entry:

Lumby, Judy, 1938– .
    Who cares?: the changing health care system.

    Includes index.
    ISBN 1 86508 056 X.

    1. Nursing—Australia. 2. Nursing—Study and teaching—
    Australia. 3. Nursing—Australia—History—20th century.
    I. Title.

610.730994

Set in 11.5/13 pt Bembo by Midland Typesetters, Maryborough, Vic.
Printed by South Wind Production Services, Singapore

10 9 8 7 6 5 4 3 2 1

CONTENTS

Acknowledgments   *vii*
Introduction   *ix*

1   The patient as informed consumer   1
2   The changing status of women   19
3   The impact of technology   36
4   The commodification of health care   54
5   The problem of equity and access   72
6   Designing health care   89
7   Major challenges   108
8   Future delivery of care   126

Conclusion   *138*
Endnotes   *145*
Index   *155*

ACKNOWLEDGMENTS

While every story is important to the storyteller, one was the initial trigger for this book. This was Sue's story which begins the book. Sue has generously included me in her story for over a decade and I thank her for that. More recently Rae and Barrie have included me in their story of diagnosis, disease and determination and glimpses of this are also between these covers.

This book has been a long time in its formulation and I acknowledge Judy Waters who first approached me to write a completely different book but was patient and enthusiastic as I wrote this one. The length of its genesis means that I owe much to the many people who have shared their stories of illness and the care they received in the system. While some of these stories are retold here, many provide a background for the issues of concern raised in the various chapters. Those support groups who generously spoke at length with me, clarifying many of the issues to do with equity and access, revealed a system which has a long way to go. The narrators are anonymous not because they necessarily asked to be but because personal details are just that—personal. Many are receiving ongoing care in the system they have critiqued.

I would also like to acknowledge my nursing and medical colleagues who gave generously of their time to discuss and debate issues with me. Those who stand out are the nurses at Concord Repatriation General Hospital who provided me with a reality check if I wandered too far away from the real world of health care. Key characters such as Ethel Lane and Professor Jim Lawrence, in particular, have so freely shared their wisdom and friendship.

This book could be criticised because of its emphasis on patients and professionals in the bush. I don't apologise for this. As I travelled around collecting stories I was amazed at the way in which nurses and patients managed alone with such little support in the most isolated of places. And they do so with little recognition. The nurses don't consider that the job they do is anything but ordinary, but the communities they care for tell another story. In writing their stories I hope to make public what is so often hidden from view in the drama of life in city hospitals.

Finally, I would like to acknowledge my friends who have lived with me being unavailable for so long. And my mother whose health became increasingly compromised over the last few years and whose death in John Hunter Hospital provided me with a story of the very best of today's health care.

My daughters and their partners continue to provide me with inspiration and support and all have been involved with the writing of this book. Alison and David shared their stories and their support and Catharine generously lent her experience and talent, despite a baby and a new job. But it is Carrie who has been with me throughout the project—sometimes supporting, more often providing harsh but well deserved critique. Thanks Carrie for getting me there.

Judy Lumby
February 2001

INTRODUCTION

It's living with the uncertainty of it all. The not knowing. Not knowing how much more life I have to live; not knowing if I might get cancer; not knowing if I might reject. And while I am grateful I had another chance ten years ago, what happens is that you spend your life living with uncertainty. After all, I had come to terms with dying and even prepared my family; then suddenly, I was offered a new chance at life. The down side of the transplant is living every day with uncertainty and medical intervention through drugs and blood tests. But you should see my wonderful garden— the daffodils are out and I have a new golden ash to plant. I just hope I live long enough to see it grow.

Sue made these remarks to me in a recent conversation—one of many we have had since she was diagnosed with a life-threatening illness. Her initial call to me followed her diagnosis with primary biliary cirrhosis, a progressive disease of unknown aetiology, and the subsequent medical directive to 'go home and get on with life—put all of this behind you'. Her first words to me were: 'I have just been told to go home and live until I die.'

Sue's story embodies so much of the best and worst aspects of our Australian health care system today. It is a paradigm for the type of medical miracles and the ethical dilemmas accompanying such miracles that occur on a daily basis. Sue's story illustrates perfectly the changing place of patients in the system. As sophisticated technology makes possible medical interventions once only imagined, the health care industry faces a whole new world: of ethical debates about who to treat and what to fund;

of resource distribution dilemmas across the health sectors; of education of specialists for new specialties; of the need to justify new techniques and practices economically; of meeting the demands of the public; and of litigation.

Despite the fact that many more lives can now be saved and life expectancy for most of us is higher than ever before, people still die and health care professionals still make mistakes. It could even be said that the health care system is now more risky than in the past because of the increased complexity of procedures, the increased toxicity of drugs and treatments, and the sicker patients who are entering the system. Despite the apparent certainty which medical science creates, the human element of fallibility remains. The diagnosis of illness and disease is unreliable because it is so dependent on human factors of time, place, practitioner and patient.

Sue's diagnosis had been quite some time in coming. Years before the diagnosis she suffered severe itching which went away. When the itch returned several years later, she had treatment from a general practitioner and a skin specialist before seeking further specialist advice. Little did she know as she gradually turned a bright orange, and lost weight, energy and hope that recent developments in medical technology would allow her another chance at life. Sue fell ill in the early days of the National Liver Transplant program at one of the largest teaching hospitals in NSW. The manufacture of the immunosuppressant drug Cyclosporin, which minimised rejection, was one of many factors which made transplantation possible. Sue was in the right place at the right time. Many things came together for this 'miracle' to occur—technology being just one of them. To survive such a life-threatening illness, of course, involves factors beyond the actual operation—things that Sue had on her side. Things such as individual tenacity, social support, faith, hope, personal control and luck, to name but a few. She was acutely aware of the circumstances under which a matching liver would become available to her, as were other transplant recipients I interviewed:

> I realised what the implications were for me to survive and I
> knew that there would have to be a tragedy for another family.
> I can remember feeling guilty when I found myself listening over

Easter for accidents. It is one thing to lose someone you love but it is another thing to be then asked to donate organs from your loved one's body.

For Sue, the first year following her transplant was more difficult than the year when she was preparing to die. Some of this was due to the physical aftermath of such long and complicated surgery, such as loss of memory—'My brain does not function the way it used to . . . it is the most frustrating thing post-transplant because I always had such a good memory and relied on it'—but it was also due to losing her career. As she told me: 'I wondered about staying alive. I resented the experience I had had because it destroyed my career path and destroyed the things that were known to me. I felt bitter about that and even thought that dying would not have been so bad.'

Readjusting to life after surgery was extremely difficult, not only for Sue but also for the many people around her. While Sue wanted to put the disease behind her, others wouldn't let her, always thinking of her (and even referring to her) as 'a liver transplant'. Having prepared for her to die, her family had to readjust to the fact that she was alive and (relatively) well. Sue had also gone through a long process of adjusting to the reality of death. She had 'stopped reading medical texts and begun to read the Bible . . . it gave me more hope'. Even facing the transplant Sue was fully prepared to die: 'Had I not come back alive I still felt that I had lived to the best possible limits and I was prepared for death—a planned funeral, a new will, and having spoken to each of my children about their future.'

Almost ten years later I received another dramatic phone call from Sue: 'I've got lymphoma. I don't want to die, I've been through so much to live.' Ironically, Sue developed this form of cancer as a direct result of the drugs she was required to take after her liver transplant. Following reduction of her immunosuppressant therapy the lymphoma size reduced but Sue began to show signs of rejecting her liver. Thus began a balancing act which continues today and which led to the conversation which began this story.

Sue is one of many individuals living with uncertainty because they have undergone and survived miraculous medical techniques,

techniques that save lives but do not necessarily have answers for their effects on survivors and their families. Indeed, Sue's story symbolises many of the complexities of health care in our nation today. Advances in technology enable lives to be saved but they require massive amounts of money to support machinery, drugs, specialist staffing, specialist units, and research and teaching funds. Industries are created to support such endeavours, industries which are difficult to dismantle. New forms of specialisation develop, in turn creating additional demand for the services they provide, which in turn raises public expectation. Subsidiary industries are created by these new technologies, in the case of transplantation for example, that of seeking donor organs. The procurement and transport of organs has created one more level of expertise, another group of specialists, technicians and protocols, all demanding funding and, of course, a new level of complexity in ethical debates.

This book has been many years in the making since it is the result of a lifetime of working in the health care system. My career as a nurse began with apprenticeship training. I continued to nurse and teach nurses while bringing up my three daughters in the 1960s and 1970s, and in the 1980s I found myself heading up one of the first departments of nursing in a College of Advanced Education. Four years later, I headed up a school of nursing in a university before moving, in the mid-1990s, into a clinical chair of nursing in a large teaching hospital. My present position as Executive Director of the NSW College of Nursing ensures my continuing involvement in a health care system which, in many ways, looks very different from the one I entered all those years ago but which, in real terms, has changed very little when it comes to the structures and power struggles.

In the main, the system continues to serve those who work in it rather than the people it is set up to care for. This realisation is what sparked my interest in trying to see the phenomena of health and illness from a patient's point of view—something that the system is not set up to recognise. The patients' narratives I have collected over many years tell the real story of what it is like to be sick, frightened and vulnerable, to feel out of control and at the mercy of others. I heard many such stories daily as I cared for people of all ages with a variety of illnesses and concerns. But they were stories that were so often ignored when it came to decision-making and treatment. While there has been some turn-around in listening to patients, their perspectives are still not given enough credence in many situations.

The years since I first put on my student's pinstriped uniform and white apron have been filled with enormous social changes, particularly for women. When I left school, the professional choices for most middle-class women were nursing or teaching. We had no university in my home town and university education was not generally part of our expectations, whatever our academic capability. Today, the choices for educated middle-class women such as my daughters are unending, and for nurses, university education has opened up a range of opportunities I would never have dreamed of. No longer are girls leaving school to automatically assume handmaiden style jobs.[1] In 1995, more girls were staying on to Year 12 than boys, and increasing numbers of women are university educated. Moreover, women today have far greater control over their reproductive years—one of the greatest breakthroughs. There has also been an improvement in women's economic independence with increasing numbers of women being the main breadwinners, up from 21 per cent in 1985 to 33 per cent in 1995. A recent report predicted that in ten years women will outnumber men as owners of small businesses in NSW.[2] Of course, much is still to be done in terms of gender equality, with only 4 per cent of women in management positions and a mere 15.5 per cent in our federal parliament in 1996.[3]

While Australian society at large is very different from the one in which I grew up, the culture of the health care system remains, in many ways, very much unchanged from that in which I trained. In particular, hospitals remain rigidly hierarchical: management and decision-making generally still do not involve those delivering care at the bedside; the system still privileges the medical profession over all others.

Of course, there are many overt changes in terms of function. Hospitals today are focused on acute care, with mainly specialist practitioners and specialist units filled with specialist technology and technicians, unlike the general hospitals of the past where the units were numbered, not named. General practitioners are now specialists in their own right, replacing the general physicians who have all but disappeared. Nurses identify themselves through the specialty in which they work, as I did myself after completing one of the first intensive care courses in the early days of intensive care units. Technology is key to much of this change. The machine has become an extension of the body, moving the carer one more step away from the sick person.

Ironically, these dramatic changes are happening in a system that has changed minimally in terms of structures, vested interests, ideologies and decision-making. Strict hierarchies still exist, just as they did when I nursed in the 1960s. While the faces and names have changed, decision-making committees are largely set up in the same way with the same groups. While there has been a gradual infiltration by others, and even by the occasional consumer, such participation is mainly tokenistic in terms of equity of representation. It is certainly true that there are units, practices and contexts where things have changed, where individuals and teams are making a difference and where the old hierarchies have been broken down and new models established. But this is far from widespread and indeed is still rare enough to be considered out of the ordinary. The main examples, in my experience, occur where disciplinary boundaries have disappeared and doctors, nurses and therapists are working as a team, with the patient's needs determining the functioning of that team. Such team work is, I would argue, integral to delivering adequate and appropriate care in the future, as is the involvement of consumers in decision-making, not only about their own health but also about the health priorities of a society which demands new structures and models of funding and care.

In this book I have tried to address the tensions which exist in this complex system with the somewhat paradoxical name of health care—a system which continually juggles the vested interests and traditional ideals of medicine (to cure), nursing (to care) and science (to discover and make progress) with those of the patients. As William May points out, most books about being ill are written either from a medical standpoint or by medical ethicists in an analytical and even dictatorial style.[4] While these approaches are certainly valid, it is, I believe, also important to try to portray the experience of illness from the patient's point of view in as concrete a way as possible.

This book is built on the stories I have heard over three decades—stories about how people stay healthy and how they manage when they become ill and even disabled. Despite their individuality, from these stories some general themes do emerge. For example, patients often talk about their need to be in control even at the time of death. These stories offer a window into the health care system, a system that often fails the individual and/or the family at crucial times.

This book can in no way address all of the issues and problems that arise out of something as complex as a national health care system. What it does is introduce the patient's voice into the debate—a debate that has conventionally largely involved politicians, doctors, sociologists and journalists. Over many years as a nurse and as a researcher focused specifically on the experience of patients in the health care system, I have been privy to patients' most intimate stories and secrets. This experience has provided me with a wealth of knowledge, as has working in the system. This book asks: what was the experience of being sick in the past, and what is it like for patients today? Is access to hospital and community care radically different in the 1990s? And what about those responsible for the care—what are the differences in terms of the way they are prepared for working in health care and in the way they interact with each other and patients? Finally, what values drive our health care system, and do we have a system that cares?

The book includes anecdotes of my own and others but the focus is firmly on the storytellers I have listened to over decades— on the stories of those who feel sick, are diagnosed as ill, are categorised with a disease, and who manifest symptoms which require investigation. When I began nursing, these people were called 'patients', during the 1970s they were termed 'customers', the 1980s was the era of the 'client', and the 1990s was the era of the 'consumer'. There is, however, a trend in the new millennium to return to the past and to the person called 'patient' or even 'person who is ill'. For the purposes of this book they will be called patients, the name that ordinary people and some professionals have always used.

This book is not just *about* patients—it is written from the patients' perspective. They speak through various sources including direct interview, anecdotes and observations. And it is intentionally written in a style that they can access. These stories are also supplemented by the insights of health care experts. Indeed, it could be said that all the stories are told by experts in their own field: the patients in the field of being ill, and the professionals in the field of their practice. Like any other, this approach has its limitations. For example, when using case studies of the past along with examples from the present, it is important to acknowledge the problematic nature of hindsight. While hindsight or recall can use the past to revise the present, it also runs the risk of distortion.[5]

The book is not offered up as an empirical study of patient experience, although it draws from such studies. In light of this, the various stories here aren't intended to provide a single 'truth' about the history of health care but rather to provide snapshots of particular patients' experiences of health care delivery over time. It aims to present, as directly as possible, the stories of people faced with a disruption to their 'normal' pattern of health. These stories are supplemented by those of professionals to provide the reader with a more comprehensive picture of the context in which patients find themselves. To be able to sketch such a picture it is also necessary to contextualise historically a number of related issues which provide the themes for each of the chapters: the political (in essence, economic) decisions which determine the mega-structures and resources; the social changes which necessarily impact on all social institutions; the changes in scientific knowledge which alter the way in which the ill person is understood, constructed and treated; and the power struggles which define the quality of care that patients receive.

Professor Jim Lawrence, an eminent physician, recently spoke to me of the qualities he thinks are necessary when practising good medicine, ones which involve a focus on the patient's perspective:

> I think it's tremendously important as a physician where your primary responsibility is mainly diagnostic which leads to therapy, to be able to communicate properly. And that means being able to communicate properly with the patient and with other sources of information which go along with the patient . . . Because if

you can't put your empathy in the context of knowledge then it's too easy to be polarised into being a totally empathetic doctor or a totally working knowledge-based, action-based doctor. And the real answer has to be a marriage of the two that is appropriate.

It is in the spirit of Professor Lawrence's comments that this book takes up the fundamental issues and problems of the Australian health care system through the stories of the patients who have had to negotiate such a complex and sometimes less than adequate system.

1

—

THE PATIENT AS INFORMED CONSUMER

When I practised as a nurse in the 1960s, patients knew so little about their condition they were often unable to explain their surgical scars. When questioned about an operation they often said things like: 'I had my insides removed.' Forty years ago, there was an overwhelming trust in doctors and nurses, as well as in the health care system itself. Complaints were rare. Those that came were made by letter after discharge and usually related to the temperature of the meals rather than to the competence of the staff. Patients' charts were kept at the desk to be read only by the charge nurse and the doctors. The one person who was never given access to the information was the patient. But this was rarely an issue.

As a nurse, I struggled with having to withhold information from patients. I felt extreme conflict about continuing to care for someone who was the only one who didn't know they were terminally ill, and about what to do when a patient I was nursing asked the dreaded question: 'What were the *real* results of the operation? Come on, you can tell me.' There were always patients who intuitively knew they had terminal cancer and a few who even spoke about the conspiracy of silence surrounding their illness. But these patients felt enormous pressure to go along with the conspiracy, even in the face of their desire to share feelings, frustrations and hopes.

Over the past forty years things have changed dramatically. Despite resistance from some in the medical profession, patients' records are now available to patients through the federal *Freedom of Information Act* (FOI) which came into force in 1982. The NSW *Freedom of Information Act* was passed in 1989 providing access to documents held by state departments and authorities. In most cases surgical patients and their families are now offered educational information and counselling sessions. As soon as possible after an operation, the majority of surgeons speak frankly to the patients and their families about the surgery and its outcomes. Except in rare cases, surgeons speak directly to the patient, not only about finding malignancies, but also about their prognosis and choices for therapy.

Not that the bare facts are all that matter. My own research into liver transplant recipients revealed that the language doctors use when they break bad news, along with their attitude when delivering the prognosis, is very important. One patient spoke to me of being given a prognosis of End Stage Liver Disease at a time when she was alone, with no support, and then having to make her way home to inform her children and parents. In the same breath the doctor had told her to 'Go out and get on with life since it may be ten years'. While this doctor certainly shared information, it was his manner and timing which required attention. Many patients who were diagnosed with terminal illnesses also spoke to me of the power of language in determining how they felt about their prognosis. They viewed 'terminal' as a term which embodied hopelessness and preferred instead 'life-threatening' which, they believed, at least offered a glimmer of hope.

In my experience as a researcher, it is common for patients and their relatives to express anger at the inadequate way health care professionals, particularly doctors, have communicated with them.

This chapter will focus on what amounts to one of the most significant changes in health care since the 1960s: the emergence of a more informed and articulate public and, therefore, patient population. Increasingly, the plethora of problems with the health care system have been exposed and discussed in popular discourse via the media, resulting in widespread disillusionment with conventional health care and medical practices. The passive role which, by and large, patients played in the 1960s has undergone a transformation to one of active participant. Or has it?

FROM PASSIVE PATIENT TO ACTIVE CONSUMER

While writing this book I visited C in her rural cottage. Her severely disabled son sat in a purpose-built chair watching television and listening to his favourite music. C spoke of the way she was treated by a doctor who spoke to her after she discovered her son had a chronic degenerative condition:

> Graham (the local doctor) had had a heart attack and he got a locum in . . . and this fellow didn't have any children and he's sitting in the chair and I walked in and he said, 'Stick him in a home and forget about him'. And his words were, 'Why bust your guts with a child like this when you've got others at home' . . . and I flew up and I said, 'How dare you speak to me like this' . . . and I walked out.

This woman, spurred on by the anger she felt at how she and her son had been treated by the medical profession, had gone on not only to care for her son at home but to set up a national support group for others in her situation.

C's frustration with her doctor, as well as her proactive approach to her son's illness, illustrates perfectly the shifting attitude of many people in the community towards the health care system. This change in public attitude has resulted in the implementation of a number of government initiatives which focus on the rights and needs of health care consumers. One of the more controversial moves, with regard to the inclusion of patients in decisions about health care delivery, has been the establishment of Health Care Complaints Units or bodies in most states. The Complaints Unit set up in NSW in 1984 met strong resistance from many professional bodies, some of which are still critical of what they see as its role in undermining professional authority. In contrast, the previous NSW Commissioner, Merrilyn Walton, understands the Complaints Unit, not as promoting one group at the expense of another (patients over doctors), but rather as simply providing a mechanism for ensuring public accountability. In addition, the *Patients' Bill of Rights* is now prominently displayed on hospital walls and lawyers openly solicit disgruntled patients. Litigation rates have increased as patients assert their rights to appropriate care of the highest standard.

3

Patients themselves are also much more likely to seek out information independently of their doctors. I recently attended a workshop set up by a group called the Consumer Focus Collaboration whose aim is to strengthen the focus on consumers in health service planning, delivery, monitoring and evaluation in Australia. At the workshop a doctor spoke of patients who came to him armed with the latest information printed off the World Wide Web along with a provisional diagnosis of their illness.

B, a senior pharmacist, talks of the 1960s and how it was for patients then and now:

> It is quite interesting. When I started, patients didn't even know what tablets they were taking but now patients come in knowing the drugs they want prescribed. It has meant a difference in access for patients but it has also meant that we (the pharmacists) are no longer, and doctors are no longer the keepers of the secrets. The doctor–patient relationship is changing as well. The legislation around Consumer Medicine leaflets and their requirement eventually by law (2002) means that drugs will have to have accompanying Consumer Medicine Information leaflets which will continue to expand the consumer's knowledge. At the moment there is still no legal obligation on the doctors, nurses or pharmacists to hand these out but many of the pharmaceutical companies have tested these with consumers. This is all to do with consumer rights. The other change has been with the Internet. Consumers are now coming in and saying to the doctor 'I want this drug' because it has been on the Internet.

What is it that has brought about this seemingly radical shift from passive patient to active consumer? While it is not possible to disentangle the causes from the effects of such an attitudinal shift, it is possible to identify some cultural and political forces which have contributed to it.

The most obvious cultural change to coincide with the shift in patient attitude since the 1960s is, of course, the accelerated proliferation of information via the mass media. Between the 1960s and the turn of the century, the amount of information about medical matters such as the body and its functioning, diseases, their causes and cures, has increased exponentially. In the

1960s, medical information was contained between the covers of medical texts, and access to it was limited to those trained to understand the specialised language of such literature. Newspapers and the few magazines available rarely addressed medical issues in any informed way. Even if such information had been available, there would have been a limited market for it because of the absolute faith placed in the family doctor as provider of all medical wisdom. Today the media dispenses up-to-date medical research findings and the latest cure-all and technological breakthroughs which enable life to be prolonged or enhanced.

And it isn't just the scope of the information that is now so readily available which has had an impact on patient expectations. It is the way it is presented: in a user-friendly, non-specialist manner, which can be easily understood by the lay person. Entire television programs are dedicated to health issues, medical debates, and stories about people's experiences with the health care system, both positive and negative. And via talk-back radio, people are willing to expose their private illnesses as well as their interactions with the health care system.

Likewise, there has been an interesting shift in advertising from the advertisements of the past which used doctors as experts, to current advertisements where the 'expert' is now the patient. Personal stories are also readily available in many popular texts, with well known personalities and ordinary people speaking out about their encounters with a variety of illnesses including cancer, Parkinson's disease and AIDS. 'How-to' magazines also focus on all aspects of how to stay healthy and offer easy-to-understand information about modern and traditional therapies.

Doctors have also assisted in the demystification of their discipline. One outstanding example is the work of Oliver Sacks, a leading neurologist best known for his books such as *The Man Who Mistook His Wife for a Hat*. His personal experiences form a vital part of each of his books, making them accessible and interesting as well as credible. A number of doctors now write weekly columns for popular magazines, while others take part in radio and television programs. Such exposure has served the medical profession well publicly by altering the perception that they are unattainable and elitist. Despite this, there is still great resistance to increased dialogue with the public from the more conservative

5

element of the medical profession, for whom a more informed patient population amounts to a direct threat to their once universal authority.

Another, but much less apparent, factor driving the shift in patient expectations is the urgent need for governments to find ways of curtailing medical costs. Although it is undoubtedly the case that certain government initiatives have been driven by popular demand, it is also true that encouraging the consumer to question services, costs and outcomes has conveniently coincided with increased pressure on government to rein in health care spending. This is particularly so in the area of acute (hospital) care. In other words, the rise in consumer participation marries with the political agenda of contemporary governments.

A good example is the establishment of the Women's Health Nurse in the 1970s. While largely a result of an overwhelming demand by women who wanted access to women-centred services delivered by women, it also provided an effective method of cost-cutting and even cost shifting from acute services to the community. Multipurpose women's health centres were conducted by female nurses, thus providing more cost-effective and efficient health care delivery, since all staff, including the doctors, were paid the same rates due to the collective nature of the centres. (This equality of pay has since changed and rates of pay are now in line with professional rates.) Many women's health nurses, who are highly specialised and experienced, saw women's health centres as opportunities to provide total health care, including education and counselling. The nurses provided advice about child rearing and general family matters. Accordingly, prevention became a major part of their role, further avoiding costly intervention and reducing government costs.

In addition to such initiatives, governments have also actively encouraged consumer participation in the health care system decision-making processes through a range of formal mechanisms. The NSW Health Care Complaints Commission, established following a review of the *Health Care Complaints Act* in 1996–97, is gradually gaining acceptance by most professional bodies. The original Health Complaints Units were established because of public disquiet about their own protection from professional indifference or negligence. And they have also been an effective mechanism for raising the awareness of health care professions and professionals about the need for accountability at all levels of care, from the initial consultation throughout the trajectory of illness. The various committees set up to investigate the quality of services (including practices) around the country are also government initiatives. Examples are the NSW Ministerial Advisory Committee on Clinical Quality and more recently the Australian Council for Safety and Quality in Health Care[1] on which consumers have a strong voice. While it is the case that such initiatives have sometimes been driven by popular demand, they have also suited a broader, sometimes contradictory, political agenda.

This political desire to implicate the patient in a more active way in health care has effected a change in the nature of the health professional–patient relationship. In particular, the strength of the consumer (patient) movement has in many ways had a significant effect on the way in which health care professionals understand their roles, particularly in relation to patients. Doctors and nurses have had to rethink their professional relationships—relationships which were previously defined as objective and distant. They can no longer pay lip service to the rights of patients as vital players in terms of their health care management (I discuss this shift in the doctor–patient relationship in more detail later in this chapter.) There is now considerable pressure on health care professionals to ensure that the process of dealing with patients and their families is a more consensual one. And political imperatives have been introduced to ensure compliance by health professionals, such as the development of indicators and the benchmarking of episodes of care which enable measurement of competence and quality service delivery to compare data across health care areas and specialists.

Evidence-based practice is one recent example of this push for professional accountability. It insists that doctors base their practice on up-to-date evidence of efficacy, a difficult ask in a world where such evidence may take years to surface in peer-reviewed publications. In the 1997–98 Federal Budget, Dr Michael Wooldridge, the Minister for Health and Family Services, described the evidence-based approach to medicine as 'the single most important line of thought over the next decade in health care management'. Wooldridge went on to claim that, as well as promoting quality of care, evidence-based medicine would 'promote cost containment because by supporting what we know works well and discouraging what we know doesn't work patient care will be more effective and we can have better cost control in a manner acceptable to the profession'. Subsequently, Wooldridge has set up the Medical Services Advisory Committee to provide advice on what will be funded or not funded under the Medicare Benefits Schedule. Insisting on scientific evidence for all new procedures or investigations has, therefore, the potential to radically reduce massive costs in areas such as pathology and radiology.

This move to justify practice through best scientific evidence rather than ritual, collegiality or tradition is not only driven by the needs of government. As I have already suggested, patients themselves are demanding the justification of a procedure, a drug or a choice in treatment. Whereas previously the management of a patient's illness was most likely to be left solely in the hands of the professionals who were perceived to have absolute expertise and knowledge, now the expertise of the health care professional is more likely to be questioned and alternatives sought. In fact, the very notion of what constitutes health has, through increased public awareness of issues not only concerning medicine but also of related fields such as psychology, been reconceptualised in popular discourse and, therefore, by patients themselves.

THE CHANGE IN PUBLIC PERCEPTION OF HEALTH

The concepts *health* and *illness* are, of course, not immutable but are constructed culturally and historically. In turn, these constructs structure the way health and illness care are delivered and, therefore, received. For example, whereas most Western countries traditionally have focused their notions of health care around illness, specifically acute illnesses, other cultures, such as the Chinese, focus on staying healthy. The way a culture funds its health care reflects its perceptions of health and illness and vice versa.

Health is currently defined by the World Health Organization (WHO) Constitution as being a 'state of complete physical, mental and social well being and not merely the absence of disease or infirmity'.[2] This general definition of health reflects current popular notions of health in the West. As the threat of epidemics lessened and advances in science enabled mass immunity from certain infectious diseases at the same time as nutrition and sanitation improved, people in developed economies began to broaden their views of illness and health. They were able to envisage a life longer and healthier than that of their mothers and fathers and, as a result, they began to rethink the very notion of what constituted a healthy life. It was a conception of health which moved beyond the mere absence of disease. As a result, the late twentieth century witnessed a new focus on mental/ emotional health. Indeed, psychological well-being is now considered an essential part of being healthy.

R, a 60-year-old Australian woman recently discharged from a private hospital after a prolonged illness, spoke to me about what health means to her. Her comments sum up the contemporary, popular, Western understanding of health prevalent in Australia today: 'I don't see that [health] as purely a medical thing. To me, being healthy is how I'm perceiving life, how I'm relating to people, how I'm coping with day-to-day things. And I guess there are more things that influence that than the physical condition of your body.'

This broader view of health stands in stark contrast to the acute-illness focus of our health care system and, in particular, to the distribution of health care funding. Increasingly, a large proportion of health care funding is spent on acute illness, particularly on surgical interventions. As a result, there is little left for the implementation and nourishment of public health strategies needed so badly to improve the basic health of disadvantaged groups such as indigenous Australians. The first research paper of the National Health Strategy (in 1992) investigated inequalities in the basic health of different groups in the community.[3] It showed that 'people with the most limited economic resources experience poorer health as measured by standardised death rates and measures of illness'. This group, because of their poorer health, are higher users of primary and secondary health services but lower users of preventive services. Tailor-made public health strategies addressing all aspects of a healthy environment, including housing, sanitation, nutrition, education and employment, are desperately needed by such groups.

As a result of the lack of resources allocated to primary health care, the public are increasingly taking it upon themselves to manage their own health and welfare. Self-medication is increasing, along with a growing awareness and acceptance of preventive medicine, and of what keeps an individual healthy. Today, we often share intimate information about our bodies and our health in our daily conversations, comparing diets, sleeping and exercise patterns, and levels of stress. Such conversations were rare in the 1950s.

Sitting on the veranda of the local museum in a rural town, D spoke to me about his days as a stockman and how he kept healthy. 'If you worked before ... you didn't need to exercise. Now you go to work and come home and do exercise.' Now not as fit and with several chronic illnesses, he spoke with humour and scepticism about the rules recently laid down for him for keeping healthy:

> I'm fit as anything. I cough a lot ... but that's where I get my exercise ... The doctor told me I should do some walking ... I took a block of wood from the pub and put it outside my door and I tell the doctor I've been round the block and he says, 'Yes, you have improved'.

Despite the resistance of people like D, however, health care professionals in rural areas, in keeping with their urban counterparts, are reporting an increased interest in health issues within the community. The local nurse of D's rural town spoke to me about the changes in the rural community she services, where research has shown poorer health statistics than those of the city. In her experience, people are becoming increasingly interested in information about how to stay healthy and much of her time is now spent conducting education programs relating to 'lifestyle' issues like smoking and drinking, diet and exercise, as well as self-management skills such as self-checks for breast and prostate cancer. As she observes:

> Men are asking me about more information ... there's a much freer rapport that I have with them ... quite a few men have said they have actively sought health checks from their GPs. I think

the general awareness . . . is growing but also there is a growing awareness in the community altogether . . . literature coming out now aimed at men about their health. There are books that you can buy. Also the fact that people are becoming freer to talk about their problems too.

What this nurse is describing is the increasing desire of the general public to take charge of their own health and well-being. Particularly since the early 1980s there has been an emphasis on, indeed obsession with, health and fitness—and health and well-being have become big business. Exercise is now one of our largest industries as joggers pound the streets with the latest equipment, expensive personal trainers become increasingly popular, and gymnasiums promise weight loss, weight gain, weight redistribution and happier, more successful lives, all for an annual fee. Pharmaceutical companies bombard us with new and better vitamin/mineral compounds in which the secret to longevity is supposedly contained. Food is dissected to within an inch of its organic components, categorised and labelled accordingly. We can buy it fat-free, chemical-free, preservative-free, sugar-free, kilojoule-free, and taste-free.

The recent demand for perfect health (and the perfect body) has created whole new job categories. Fitness trainers, lifestyle managers, beauty therapists and psychic gurus have capitalised on and helped to manufacture our obsession with our bodies. In the USA this has reached manic proportions with the restructuring, reorganising and reorientation of people becoming a huge industry. Bodies are now manufactured, manipulated and managed. The ultimate medical manipulation of our bodies is, of course, plastic surgery. Advertising constantly bombards us with messages concerning our ability to reinvent our own bodies through diet, exercise and surgery. As a cultural medium, our bodies are also regulated by norms perpetuated through these media images. The advertising associated with the commodification of our well-being has impacted both positively and negatively. While providing a vector for the dissemination of information, it has also increased the anxiety and confusion we have about avoiding illness (and perhaps even death) and having the perfect life and body.

But despite this popular focus on health, the system which we call the 'health' care system is, more than ever, focused on illness. Between 1996 and 1997/98 there was a 2.3 per cent increase in hospital admissions, despite the negligible rise in available hospital beds in that time.[4] This was possible because length of hospital stay decreased to allow for higher turnover of surgical patients through the system, including an increase in day only patients of 6.4 per cent in the same period. Apart from the occasional rehabilitation gymnasium attached to a hospital, there is little attempt to link the public focus on health and well-being into the health care system. In truth, we are operating an illness care system. Our priorities for funding, our models of care and the power structures inherent in the system all reflect this. *Health* has little to do with any of what goes on in hospitals. Patients are rarely discharged 'well'. They are usually recuperating from surgery and may even have a hospital-acquired infection or have suffered an adverse event.[5] Not all patients in hospitals are there for surgical intervention, but all have an illness which is considered life-threatening since this was the criterion for admission to a public hospital in 1999.[6]

In the past, patients remained in hospital until they were mobile, pain-free and organised about their long-term care, but this is no longer the case. There are valid reasons for moving patients on, like the fact that hospitals are dangerous places due to infection and patients run the risk of being 'medicalised' the longer their stay. But patients still require adequate follow-up in the community to ensure infection-free wounds, correct drug regimes (particularly for pain), and support with long-term outcomes of surgery such as stomas and so on. Services in the community have not been funded to cope with these changes. The responsibility for follow-up care has increasingly shifted to the patient and their loved ones.

Accordingly, the general public have become much more likely to seek alternatives to those offered by conventional medicine. One of the most significant consequences of the contemporary focus on physical, mental and emotional well-being and the growing disillusionment with the conventional system has been the increasing rejection of conventional medicine and medical practices in favour of what are termed 'alternative' therapies. These so-called alternatives are in fact traditional therapies ousted when modern medicine gained its scientific foothold in the mid-1800s. Australian research has shown that 50 per cent of people seeking modern medical treatments are backing this up with alternative treatments.[7] Up to 80 per cent of the population worldwide rely on what we would regard as alternative medicine as their primary mode of health care, so what may be unusual for us is routine health care for this 80 per cent. As far as Australians are concerned, we spend up to $900 million a year on so-called 'complementary treatments'.[8]

The treatments that are becoming increasingly popular include acupuncture, homeopathy, iridology, hypnotherapy, naturopathy, aromatherapy, and herbs. These have been incorporated into many people's lives for some time now as daily routines. Alternative therapies now account for $900 million outlay per year in Australia. For patients who are accessing both conventional and alternative medicine, the cost of health care is doubled and nationally it increases the amount spent on health (and illness).

Recognition of traditional Chinese medicine has recently translated into registration of practitioners and universities offering undergraduate and postgraduate degrees. Patients with illnesses such as autoimmune disorders, irritable bowel syndrome, cancer, arthritis, infertility, and even asthma are the most likely to consult such practitioners because they are often unable to be treated successfully by conventional medicine. There are also those who attend as a preventive measure and those who simply want to optimise their feeling of well-being.

A senior health care professional I interviewed spoke of her own experience of rejecting, in frustration, conventional medicine in favour of 'alternative' treatment. She underwent an extremely expensive arthroscopy for a chronically damaged knee, which left her even more incapacitated than before. The surgeon's parting remarks didn't instil much faith either: 'I'll see you in a few months for a knee replacement.' Frustrated because of her immobility and pain, she sought alternative therapy in the form of acupuncture. A year later, not only does she now have a knee which can function but she is pain-free and mobile, with no apparent need for further intervention. She regularly refers people to her Chinese acupuncturist for a variety of problems, many of who have become chronic because of the inability of our health care system to deal with them.

The main barrier to more widespread acceptance of such treatment is currently the cost, since these treatments are often not adequately covered by insurance funds.

In response to this renewed popularity of 'alternative' medicine, mainstream medicine has gradually begun to incorporate traditional therapeutic practices into its repertoire. Walking down an inner suburban street recently I counted half a dozen group medical practices advertising both modern and traditional approaches. The University of Sydney, considered a traditional institution, now has a centre for herbal medicine, while the Royal Women's Hospital Nursing Centre for Women's Health has conducted a randomised control study using acupressure bands to control distress from nausea and vomiting during pregnancy and post-surgery. A Natural Therapies unit was also set up in the hospital. Pharmaceutical company Quantale Limited recently identified the potential for combining modern medicine with homeopathy and is launching a range of products. Alternative therapies are equally making inroads into modern medical courses with more than 3000 general practitioners having joined the Australian Integrative Medical Association. Nurses have long been involved in alternative therapies, with some practising independently and others integrating them into their daily practice within conventional medical contexts.

Despite these measures, the acceptance of traditional/alternative therapies within mainstream Australian medicine has been slow. Even those practitioners who have undertaken the same rigorous training as Western doctors in addition to years of learning/practising traditional Chinese medicine techniques find it hard to get recognition. The lack of evidence for traditional therapies (measured according to modern scientific methods) remains a contentious issue with the majority of practitioners in both traditions. Given the revelation in more recent times that modern medicine itself lacks scientific evidence for much of its own procedures and treatments, such objections lack consistency. I have sat through many hours of Ethics Committee deliberations regarding proposals by Chinese doctors who wanted to validate their practices through scientific research. The debate was rarely about the scientific rigour of the research but rather revealed a deep-seated suspicion of any medicine not Western in its approach.

Practices such as acupuncture and herbal medicine are increasingly being exposed to rigorous randomised trials in an effort to facilitate their acceptance by the modern medical fraternity. Recently, there has been some acknowledgment of 'alternative' practices in the publication of six studies of alternative therapies in the prestigious medical journal, the *Journal of American Medicine*.[9] It will be interesting to see how quickly and how widely such therapies are adopted into mainstream health care in this country. One can already find hospitals where massage and aromatherapy are part of mainstream nursing practice, but even within such institutions these practices are not accepted as serious therapies, but regarded more as pleasant distractions for patients (and even nurses). Nevertheless, we've come a long way from the days when I was warned about smiling and chatting with patients, let alone massaging them (although I regularly did so behind the screens!).

THE IMPACT ON THE DOCTOR–PATIENT RELATIONSHIP

As should now be clear, of all the relationships within the health care system it is the one between doctor and patient which has been affected most overtly by the shift in patients' attitudes about their health and the health professional's role in its management. No longer is the conventional medical doctor considered the universal authority on issues of health and illness. The local general practitioner, for example, no longer plays the role of father confessor who visits the home at all hours, looking after the whole family and dispensing unquestioned wisdom. The family doctor is less likely to play such a central role in the management of the family's well-being.

Dr B, a family doctor of nearly fifty years' standing, spoke to me recently about the way he had practised general medicine in his local area. His surgery, which is still being used as one of only a few general practices attached to a home, was the scene of many surgical procedures: 'Many general practices now keep routine business hours, and with few offering home visits, patients attend privately-run Medical Centres or hospital emergency units with anonymous doctors who change with each visit.'

This is not to deny that many general practitioners are working extremely long hours and are dedicated to personal contact with patients and families. But because of the structure of the Medicare rebates, they need to work harder by pushing more patients through to earn a living. There is no financial incentive for long consultations unless your practice is in a more affluent area where it is not necessary to bulk-bill. Dr Birch, a general practitioner recently profiled in a Sunday paper, spoke of 'being out of control' because of the pressure of seeing up to seventy patients a day both in the surgery as well as in their homes. He refers to the competition set up by the rise in 'superclinics' run by businessmen, open at all hours, occupying prime locations and offering convenience medicine.[10]

As I have already suggested, in parallel with these practical changes there has been a radical shift in interpersonal relations between doctor and patient. This shift has been a source of anxiety for health care professionals such as doctors whose roles in the past were defined by the passivity of the patient. The beneficence model of old was, by and large, a very comfortable one in which to work as a professional. You had control and could therefore orchestrate the relationship to your liking. Of course, in retrospect it was inappropriate in so many ways, not the least of which being the lack of acknowledgment of the patient's rights. It was as if patients had no autonomy in relation to their bodies and their illnesses. In turn, the undermining of the traditional doctor–patient relationship has provoked anxiety in many patients. While some sections of the community question doctors, many patients are happier assuming a passive role in relation to doctors. They expect a doctor to make all the decisions, including future management choices, and would be disappointed, even angry, if they were expected to be involved as an active participant in the management of their health and illness.

So, despite the claim that patients are much more assertive, I remain unconvinced that the pendulum has swung very far in terms of patients demanding control over care, specifically in relation to the doctor. If at all, it is only likely to happen after the doctor has left the ward or the patient has left the clinic. Despite the fact that there is certainly evidence of disillusionment with the medical profession among the general public, in my research

I found little evidence to support the belief that the doctor is losing status or public approval.

Increased litigation is often cited as evidence that doctors have lost their status among the general public. Yet, while it is true that there has been an increase in complaints, the hype surrounding this supposed 'explosion' has very little base in reality. Only 4 per cent of cases get to court in Australia and there is no trend towards criminalisation of professional conduct at this juncture, with the few criminal convictions being those related to doctors assaulting patients. Commenting on the medical culture of doctors protecting each other and refusing to testify against one another, Merilyn Walton notes that 'People are often reluctant to admit mistakes when they occur and often close ranks'.[11] The importance of appropriate handling of concerns before they become formal legal complaints cannot be overstated, according to Walton, who comments that 'many patients are driven to litigation because of the poor attitude of those responding to their complaints'.[12] This includes all health professionals, not only doctors.

In recognition of the communication problems between doctors and patients and the continuing reluctance on the part of patients to assert their needs, there are now a number of strategies in place which attempt to rectify some of the inherent power imbalances in the doctor–patient relationship. For example, Patient Support Officers have been appointed across seven metropolitan locations and one regional centre in NSW to address local concerns at the point of contact. Consumers can contact the officer in their particular area to request assistance as problems arise. In 1998 a pilot program of inmate patient support began in NSW Correctional Centres because this group has been identified as having difficulty accessing information and resolving health concerns.

Professor Miles Little, a retired surgeon and now Director of the Centre for Values, Ethics and the Law in Medicine at the University of Sydney, believes that medicine has lost touch with the community. As he puts it so succinctly: 'We cure more, results are better than they've ever been, life expectancy has gone up by 27 years and everybody hates the medical profession. People are profoundly dissatisfied.'

In order to redress some of this dissatisfaction, Little believes that change should occur at the very beginning of a doctor's training. He recommends the introduction of 'humane values' to medical degrees by educating students in the humanities in addition to their scientific studies. For Little and many others, a humanities education will better equip doctors for communicating with patients more effectively and more compassionately. It remains to be seen if this strategy and the many others now in place to improve doctor–patient relations will be successful.

2

THE CHANGING STATUS OF WOMEN

As a little girl I formed my image of the nurse from an educational picture book called *When I Grow Up*. The career choices described in the book were clearly sex-segregated. For a girl, the choices were nurse, secretary, hairdresser, housekeeper, mother. Secretly I coveted the choices the companion boys' book offered my brother. These included what seemed much more exciting options: a doctor replete with a white coat and stethoscope, pilot, fireman, coalminer, train driver. Not only was nursing a 'feminine' job, it was obviously categorised with the trades rather than the professions.

When I began nursing, student nurses were only one rung above cleaners in terms of status in the hospital and even then the cleaners were usually more aware of the ward politics than we were. They even counselled the patients since we, the nurses, were not allowed to engage the patients in 'small talk'. I remember being warned not to smile at the patients in a male ward as I might 'encourage' them. Given that the majority were strung up to traction with ropes and pulleys and were totally confined to their beds, I now wonder what such encouragement could lead to. I was also forbidden to speak to the doctors—interaction with the doctor was limited to the head nurse. We stood aside for doctors just as we stood aside for the head nurses, with hands behind our backs and eyes averted.

Doctors lectured to nurses in training, which reinforced these notions of obedience and subservience. It was in the interest of doctors to perpetuate this traditional understanding of the nurse—

by producing compliant nurses they were better able to maintain their own authoritative status. Showalter, citing Baumgart,[1] claimed that the nurse training regimes bore the imprint of Florence Nightingale's notoriously critical views on female ignorance, laziness, incompetence and lack of moral purpose. This hierarchy left nurses a legacy of low power roles, intense dedication and obedience— a legacy which even today spills over into community expectations of nurses.

This chapter develops some of the ideas I introduced in Chapter 1 by addressing one of the most influential changes over the past forty years: the changing status of women in Australian society. The reason for examining this social phenomenon is simple: the health care system reflects wider society in that the gendering of roles which has maintained the system is now under critique and reform as the influence of the women's movement makes it mark. Moreover, the contemporary focus on the health of specific groups can also be linked to the widespread acceptance of (at least some of) the values of the women's movement.[2]

WOMEN'S PLACE IN SOCIETY

In the 1950s and 1960s most Australian men and women took it for granted that the family was the fulcrum of society. As Rosemary Pringle notes: 'The family, understood as a self-contained unit of parents and children living as a separate household, was celebrated as the ideal form of living arrangement for the modern world.'[3]

Gender relations were organised around this family unit. Men took the primary role in the public world of work and citizenship, women were aligned with the domestic sphere of home duties and childcare.

In the 1970s, the rise of the women's movement confronted this 'natural' division of labour and identified the nuclear family as the central locus of patriarchy and a root cause of women's oppression. Issues such as domestic violence, child sexual abuse, rape in marriage, access to abortion, and the unpaid nature of women's work became key issues in the fight for women's rights. This struggle spawned women's refuges, women's health centres, rape crisis centres, and grassroots organisations aimed at changing the status of women.

The women's movement was, of course, by no means homogenous. By the mid-1970s clear factions had emerged in Australian feminism. As Wilkinson and Howard point out in *Tomorrow's Women*,[4] a major report on women in the United Kingdom, 'Tomorrow's women will be more different from each other than women are today in terms of life experience, opportunities. There will be no women's movement—only women's movements, no feminism, only feminisms.' The women's liberation movement, for example, advocated a self-consciously radical politics with a focus on protest, activism and distrust of the patriarchal state. The Women's Electoral Lobby, by contrast, had a liberal agenda. It focused on equal opportunity measures for women such as equal pay, childcare and anti-discrimination legislation. Despite the diversity which grounds the history of Australian feminism, a range of unified goals, if not unified methods, emerged from this period. These included: the enactment of the 1975 federal *Sex Discrimination Act*, the battle for equal pay which resulted in women being entitled to the same minimum wage as men, and the goal of increased access to higher education and training.

For many women born in the 1930s and 1940s, the changes were dramatic—for some, revolutionary. Women who had married young and produced children in the expectation that their lives would revolve around the family were suddenly presented with opportunities to enter the workforce or study at a tertiary institution. In 1966 only 29 per cent of married women participated in the paid workforce. And in professions such as the public service, nursing and teaching, women were required to resign on marrying. By 1975 this participation rate had grown to 41 per cent. The equal wage decision of the Commonwealth Arbitration Court in 1972 is often viewed as the turning point in women's participation, but as Deborah Mitchell notes: 'We must look to other factors to explain the growth of women's participation—especially among married women.'[5] She lists the lifting of the bar on employment of married women in the Commonwealth Public Service in 1966, federal legislation to combat employment discrimination, and increased access to education—all initiatives driven by the women's movement. As well, the increase in female educational attainment, as Mitchell notes, across the generations is remarkable. Dr Bob Birrell, a researcher at the Centre for Population and Urban Research at Monash University, found that 'In every year since 1984 more women than men have started university courses'.[6] In 1996 13 per cent more women than men aged 20–24 held degrees. Birrell's research has identified higher education as the crucial factor protecting women against poverty (single mothers are at high risk of living in poverty) and unemployment. Fifty per cent of university educated women in their early thirties are childless, compared to 30 per cent of women with no post-school qualifications.

Like all other changes in the status of women, the increased education of women has created a certain amount of anxiety. A study in the late 1970s by Dr Susan Kelly, the general manager of the NSW Council of Adult Education,[7] showed that mature aged female students had a divorce rate three times higher than that of the normal population. My own experience as an academic managing the problems of students confirms this. Mature age women lacking in confidence in the first semester would be heading the class by the end of first year. Second year would then bring a steady stream of these women into my office sharing their woes, in particular divorce threats from their partner. Kelly's longitudinal study followed these mature age women for eight years, during which profound changes were noted. They expressed the desire to 'develop an identity separate from their roles as a wife and mother'.

Despite the difficulties many married women with children faced in the transition from the role of wife and mother to student, participation in tertiary education continued to grow throughout the 1970s, 1980s and 1990s. There are a number of important related effects of education on the status of women. First, education increases potential earnings and makes joining the labour force more attractive than working at home. Second, as educational levels rise, the participation gap between men and women narrows. An early 1990s study bears this out. While three-quarters of men who left school early are in the labour force, less than half of female early leavers are. Yet, among those holding tertiary degrees, 92 per cent of men and 81 per cent of women are in the labour force. As Mitchell notes, 'This indicates that education might exert an additional influence over and above that of economic rewards: by shaping women's preferences in the choice between domestic and market labour, enhancing women's perceptions of the economic and social desirability of work, and making financial independence attainable'.[8]

It is generally assumed that the increase in educational and professional opportunities for women has achieved one of the most significant goals of the women's movement: the erosion of the gendering of professional roles. But although it is certainly true that women now have much greater access to professions previously closed off to them, it is also the case that women are still often denied access to senior positions in such professions. Moreover, professions that were traditionally considered 'feminine' have tended to remain so. The health care professions provide a good illustration of this. Traditionally, nursing was considered a female profession, medicine a male one. The exclusion of men from the early years of nurse training in Australia ensured this. And, even since the acceptance of males into nursing, the percentage of males who apply for nursing still remains relatively low (between 12 and 16 per cent)—despite the move to university education which many believed would make the profession more attractive to men. Young men entering nursing often tell me that they were actively discouraged by family and friends from undertaking nursing which is still seen as women's work.

Just as nursing was considered a female profession, so too medicine was seen as a traditionally male pursuit. In the 1950s, women in medicine were rare. By virtue of their social circumstance, women were indirectly denied access to medical degrees at universities. By the 1990s, this gender imbalance had altered considerably, although not without a struggle. In the USA the Women's Equity Action League claimed sex discrimination in a class action suit against medical schools in 1970, while in the UK an increase in the number of women entering medicine has been achieved following a 1991 Department of Health initiative for positive discrimination.

Women now constitute 50 per cent of all graduates from university medical degrees; however, this is still not reflected in women's representation in 'elite' areas of medicine. The positioning of female doctors mainly in areas outside the traditionally male areas of surgery and gynaecology, and the lack of men entering nursing despite positive campaigns, raise the question of whether the gendering of roles has really been undermined. Indeed, while it is certainly the case that there have been significant changes for women professionally in the post-war period, it is also true that there is still a long way to go to achieve equality in the workplace.

THE IMPACT OF THE WOMEN'S MOVEMENT ON NURSING

> In so many ways the challenges and difficulties that nurses have experienced in establishing access to appropriate education programs, equitable wage outcomes and proper professional recognition and career opportunities within the health care system have paralleled the same challenges and difficulties that women have faced in the wider community as they struggled and continue to struggle for true equality in all aspects of their lives.[9]

In her maiden speech to the NSW state parliament, Patricia Staunton, the ex-General Secretary of the NSW Nurses' Association, claimed the ongoing efforts to professionalise nursing provide an example of women's continuing struggle for equality generally. Indeed, as a female-dominated profession, nursing provides a unique index of the wider struggle of women to achieve equality within the workforce. As the largest professional female workforce in Australia, nursing is in fact a barometer for the changes in the status of women, particularly since the 1960s. And, because nursing as a profession is so inextricably bound up with the male-dominated profession of medicine, the medical resistance to changes in the nursing profession is instructive of the type of resistance posed by patriarchy to women's struggle for professional recognition in general.

When I began nursing in the 1960s, it was considered an appropriate and respectable job for women—a job which contributed to the good of society. It was a 'nice' thing for a young woman to do. Its tasks were domestic ones, housekeeping and nurturing. Medicine was for well brought up men, a profession

24

requiring high level skills, intelligence and an ability to command respect. The strict training regime of nursing also cultivated the 'feminine' qualities of submissiveness and obedience. This traditional image of the nurse is best reflected in this early description:

> That person alone is fit to nurse or to attend the bedside of a patient who is cool headed and pleasant in demeanour, does not speak ill of anybody, is strong and attentive to the requirements of the sick and strictly and indefatigably follows the instructions of the physician.[10]

As women in general (but not across the board) have gained a new level of confidence in their professional identities, so too have nurses begun to question their traditional roles as handmaidens for doctors. It is now clear that nurses have been held back professionally and politically by the subservience and obedience required of them. The way nursing work is managed, controlled and paid is a direct result of the way the profession has been constructed, both socially and practically, as a 'feminine' and therefore 'inferior' profession. Status, management and decision-making are the very issues which women in the wider society have had to understand and confront in an effort to gain recognition for their part in the paid (and unpaid) workforce. There is no denying that nursing has changed in status over the last two decades, primarily through changes in conditions but in particular through their move into the higher education sector. Wages and conditions have improved and career opportunities are much broader than they were when I trained. Nursing is gradually being recognised as a profession and afforded some of the advantages which go with professional status, for example, improvements in career and a voice in decision-making (although it often remains tokenistic). The changes to wages and conditions were negotiated by the Royal Australian Nursing Federation during 1988[11] with a vision of greater opportunities for nurses in all contexts and commensurate financial rewards recognising levels of knowledge and experience. However, there have been some drawbacks for the profession because of its strong historical association with trade unions, the sign of the blue-collar, unskilled worker. Whereas medicine's professional associations were identified as professional rather than industrial, allowing them to focus on 'big' issues such as the protection of professional boundaries, nursing was fighting for basic rights such as wages and conditions.

As part of this ongoing struggle, nurses have become much more involved in the politics of health care. With increased feelings of self-worth, primarily the result of increased education (to be discussed below), they are now well-placed to question decisions and decision-making practices. When I began nursing, I, like many of my colleagues, had been taught to avoid anything vaguely resembling politics. I was not raised in a household where politics was discussed in front of women and in nursing we were warned of the dangers of women becoming engaged in such 'masculine' practices. The political frame of every situation is now more obvious to most nurses, beginning at the patient's bedside and moving to meetings and clinical decisions about patient management. Deciding what is appropriate in terms of the right thing to do at this time for this patient requires the nurse to have a heightened sense of the political. My previous role as a clinical professor of nursing in a world of male professors of surgery was a political one in many ways. Increasingly, nurses are becoming more savvy in terms of 'capital P' politics. The NSW Independent Nurse Practitioner legislation is a good example, although its outcome is still uncertain and the backlash may be severe. Nevertheless, this was driven by nurses over many years; we used our honed political skills to ensure that eventually it became legislation.

Nursing's move to higher education

As with most other forms of female professional development, the single most influential factor for nursing's professionalisation and politicisation has been its move into the higher education sector. Almost overnight, nurses in NSW went from being equivalent to trade apprentices to tertiary students, a move announced by the then NSW Minister for Health Mr Laurie Brereton on 7 November 1983.[12] In 1960, nurses in Australia were trained through an apprenticeship system in which students moved through three or four years of learning on the job by copying the senior nurses. The focus of this training was the moral and spiritual development of girls rather than the development of knowledge required for safe care. In 1984, this type of hospital training was replaced with a college diploma. Two years later, when Colleges of Advanced Education were amalgamated with universities, the initial award moved to degree status. Other states followed NSW's lead so that by 1990 all nurses were educated through the university system.

Now nurses are qualified academically, many not only with undergraduate but also with postgraduate qualifications, placing them in a new political and professional position. Accordingly, nurses today are more likely to feel on a par with their professional colleagues in the health care system. This is evidenced in the way nurses are publicly questioning decisions concerning the patient, even demanding to be part of senior decision-making. The majority of state and federal working parties set up to investigate health care issues have at least one nurse representative, although we remain severely under-represented proportional to medicine. And often the committees on which nurses are invited to sit are concerned with what are perceived to be 'female' issues: services, clinical guidelines or certain ethical concerns rather than allocation of funding or structuring of service.

Nursing's move to academia was not only significant in terms of what it afforded women, it also made apparent the resistance to any change in women's status or role. The absolute furore that followed the announcement of our move into universities had little precedence in terms of media coverage. Accountancy, building and business, all male-dominated disciplines, had been transferred into universities immediately prior to nursing, with minimal fuss. There were claims that nurses were abandoning their obligations to society. After all, the very nature of nursing, the nurturing, supportive role which nurses over centuries had filled, seemed antithetical to what is popularly considered the self-interested pursuit of knowledge in academia. Nurses were considered doers not thinkers. Dr Bruce Shepherd, an orthopaedic surgeon and the then president-elect of the NSW branch of the Australian Medical Association, publicly condemned the nurse educators, in his words 'hairy-legged Stalinists', who were behind this move. While acknowledging that nurses and doctors worked as co-professionals, in the same breath Shepherd asserted that there 'could only be one boss'. The AMA (NSW) response was to announce they would be setting up their own alternative nursing program. In contrast to Shepherd's attack, Dr Anne Summers, then attached to the Federal Office of the Status of Women, spoke of this move to higher education in very different terms: as an important recognition of women's roles and rights. She referred to the fact that women in general doing the same work as men received only 78 per cent of men's earnings and that the comparable worth case conducted by the ACTU on behalf of the Royal Australian Nursing Federation was 'important for all Australian women'.[13]

It seems, then, that one way to interpret the anxiety which coalesced around nursing's move to higher education is to view it as arising primarily out of the fear that if nurses became educated they would no longer be happy performing menial tasks and deferring to doctors. In other words, it was grounded in the same type of fear that many men had about the education of women generally. It is undeniable that many professional medical bodies, but not all, have continued to be vocal critics of what nursing itself perceives to be positive changes to its profession. Individual doctors continue to express concern about the changes to nursing and nurses. Letters by doctors to newspapers about the move to recognise the role of nurse practitioners in remote and rural areas demonstrate such concerns and even fear.

> A professor of surgery once said you could train a monkey to perform an operation. To train it to correctly arrive at the decision to operate, that is the hard part. This about sums up the difference between doctors and their pretenders (nurses). Working with doctors does not make one a doctor even if it is for twenty years.[14]

This letter is written in an era when nurses work independently in rural and remote areas, diagnosing, treating and generally managing the care of many in the communities in which they work because there is no, or only limited, medical backup. It is also the era in which many nurses are both university educated and possess an extremely high level of practical experience and expertise. Not that nurses want to be doctors. However, increasingly, they do expect recognition from their medical colleagues for the skills and knowledge they possess.

It is not only medicine which has resisted change in nursing;

the public also appears either to be unaware of the changes or prefers to ignore them. By and large, they also want to believe that there will always be a group of caring, nurturing women to care for them. Despite the improvements in nurses' conditions and status, there is strong evidence that the public, to a large extent, still views nurses as no more than handmaidens to doctors. In 1989 I carried out a study to evaluate the changes in our public image as a result of registered nurses now being educated at university and graduating with a degree. Five years after our entry into higher education institutions with two classes of nurse graduates now in the workforce, I found that nurses were still perceived by the public to be stereotypically 'feminine' in character: selfless, not very well educated, obedient, and the ones who carry out the orders of the doctor.[15] And, if television is an accurate reflection of public opinion, this image was certainly alive and well at the turn of the century. Media representations of nurses fall into two dominant types: angry old matron, or sexy and available young nurse in a short uniform.

This stereotype is inevitably challenged once an individual encounters the health care system where nurses carry out the bulk of day-to-day care. This often means coordinating and negotiating across the different aspects of the patient's care to ensure that the patient is checked out by the medical team: physiotherapists or occupational therapists undertake their therapy; drugs are checked by pharmacists for likely antagonistic reactions; required procedures, tests and referrals are scheduled at appropriate times and carried out; the patient is prepared properly; the social worker has been notified of any social concerns prior to discharge; and the patient is kept informed at each stage of his/her care. It is increasingly evident to the patient that the nursing role has become more complex and difficult. Despite this, however, many nurses still feel they are treated as no more than glorified maids.

It is not surprising then that, as a result of the persistent perception of nurses as handmaidens coupled with their increased education, nurses are leaving the profession and fewer women are choosing nursing as a career option. A recent study commissioned by the NSW Health Department investigating the shortage of nurses, particularly in specialist areas, identified that 'a combination of budgetary issues, more acute patients and less staff is causing increased levels of stress and diminishing job satisfaction for all nurses'.[16] This report, which involves nurses in senior positions well qualified with many years of experience, is more telling in what is left unsaid. Professional women today, particularly university educated ones, are less likely to put up with poor working conditions and lack of recognition of their expertise and their level of responsibility. Those nurses I have interviewed who have moved careers spoke to me of now being openly valued for their contribution to their workplace, of being less stressed and of having improved work conditions.

SOME IMPLICATIONS FOR PATIENTS

How have the social and political changes effected by the women's movement impacted the day-to-day services for patients? It is possible to identify a number of changes in the types of services, attitudes of professionals, delivery patterns, funding and access—all of which affect patients and all of which have been brought about directly or indirectly as a result of the efforts of the women's movement. First, the move toward a transparent and inclusive decision-making model in health care, particularly in the last decade, has meant that a more comprehensive picture of the patient is now considered in decision-making processes. As I have already suggested, such changes have translated into more women being involved in health care decision-making processes. Certainly the consumer movement has been led chiefly by women; in the committees on which I sit, the consumer representatives are all women, and while the job has recently been vacated, the only NSW Health Complaints Commissioner has been a woman.

Despite this leadership by women and the move to a more collaborative approach within health care, it is questionable whether patients have benefited from such change. It is often assumed that the increased participation of women and the more collaborative approach to health care equate to improved conditions for patients. And it is certainly the case that some patients and their families report improvements in how they are treated. I recently interviewed a man who reflected on the differences between his experience with the health care system in the 1950s and his experience now. In the 1950s he was hospitalised for long periods with tuberculosis; more recently he encountered the system when his wife was acutely ill and hospitalised for two months. He speaks about the great changes he has personally observed in the way patients and their visitors are treated, changes he sees as for the better:

> People who were patients weren't ordered about [this time]. In the old system when you went into a hospital in the '50s you felt as if you belonged to an army group where you were told this is what you had to do, these are the rules . . . this is what you've got to do all day. If anybody stepped out of line the matron would be around to see them. I felt there was always a lot of tension between the staff and the patients. It was almost them and us . . . little groups used to get up to all sorts of pranks to upset the system then, because it was just like a form of army life. Nowadays there is a lot more compassion in the approach. It's certainly still not 100 per cent but in any sort of an operation, whether it's business or hospitals, you still find this anyway.

Despite these changes, research into patient satisfaction today demonstrates a number of significant concerns for surgical patients across five major teaching hospitals. These include issues which are assumed to have improved as a result of women's increased professional participation in the health care system and the more collaborative approach to decision-making: communication by doctors and nurses, empathy, reliability, and responsiveness of staff.[17]

The increased blurring of medical and nursing roles in the workplace has also affected the patient in many ways. New nursing positions, such as Case Managers who manage care and the proposed Nurse Practitioners in rural and remote areas, certainly place the nurse as the central negotiator with patients and their families. As I have already suggested, such moves, while often beneficial for patients, have unfortunately created tension, even harassment, in the workplace.[18] Examples of this tension include the reaction by some doctors to a questioning of their clinical decisions by nurses and their reaction to the NSW legislation enabling the development of up to forty nurse practitioner positions in rural and remote areas. While nurses in these areas have been practising in extended roles for decades, often being the only health professional in the area and unprotected by legislation, the Royal Australian College of General Practitioners (RACGP) and the AMA have strongly condemned the move. Recently the RACGP stated that they were setting up their own investigation into the nurse practitioner legislation and roll out plan. Despite the medical profession's extensive involvement at all levels in what was a six year lead-in time to this legislation, both associations attempted to impede the passage of the legislation.

How much has the campaign by the doctors affected patient care or service delivery? I suspect very little. However, some of the scare tactics in the rural areas has caused discomfort for the nurses in the present positions and disquiet for communities who do not understand what is at stake in such campaigns. Headlines in the local papers such as 'A Black Day for Rural Health' do little to instil confidence in communities who already feel disempowered in terms of access to health care services. It was necessary for the NSW College of Nursing and the NSW Department of Health to conduct a counter-campaign to clarify many questions and correct misinformation about the introduction of nurse practitioners.

One of the changes for nursing which has had an unequivocally positive affect on patient care is the new nursing career structure. There is now ensured recognition and reward for the clinician who stays at the bedside rather than moving to education and management. Patients now have access to clinical nurse consultants who are very specialised in fields such as burns, wound dressings, stomal therapy, palliative care and dialysis, to name but a few. Most of these nurses have postgraduate degrees in their speciality, and ten to fifteen years of clinical experience. One of the patients I recently interviewed, B, was particularly aware of what he described as the 'immense' changes between the nurse of the 1950s and the nurse of today:

> The nurses of the past had a lot of devotion. I think devotion
> would be on a par with what we get today. Techniques are
> certainly a lot different. The relaxed attitude they have to patients
> is another of their abilities nowadays—to be relaxed and still able

to perform the duties that they have to. I think there was a lack of knowledge with the nurses of the past . . . and the ability to work in tandem with doctors now. In the past I would never see a nurse question or even feel relaxed with some of the doctors . . . I've heard it in the corridors, more discussion with the practising medical staff who come to the hospital and the nursing staff.

Another major impact of the women's movement on the health care system has been the change in the way women are viewed within the system as patients, how they are treated, and how they demand to be treated. But, while this recognition of women's health is a seemingly positive step, there is also evidence that the focus on women's health has in fact helped to pathologise women's bodies unnecessarily. Many feminist commentators have criticised both the medicalisation of women's bodies and the gendered construction of illness. The most powerful example of this is that of childbirth. Today, many women expect medical intervention into what were once considered the 'normal' events of pregnancy and childbirth. Birth intervention rates have risen over the last decade, particularly epidurals and caesarean sections.

This increased medicalisation of women's bodies has meant big business for health care professionals and the industries attached to them. As Lovell points out:

> The treatment of women has always contributed toward the yearly income of the general practitioner, while the gynaecologist continues to fatten upon the revenue he receives from operations . . . Ovarotomies and laparotomies have become an epidemic in some localities to the extent that many surgeons think they will be branded as being unskilful if they allow their patients to get well without operative procedures.[19]

In Australia we have one of the highest rates of hysterectomy in the world. Specialists often blame this phenomenon on the women who demand such surgery, and it is, of course, not possible to attribute any single cause to the increased rates of (sometimes unnecessary) medical intervention with women's bodies. Nevertheless, it is an example of how the women's movement, in attempting to make women and their needs more visible, has had both positive and (unintended) negative effects on women as patients.

It is also commonly assumed that another significant change for patients in the health care system and brought about by the changing status of women has been the increase in female doctors. It is sometimes assumed that women will bring more 'humane' feminine values to the practice of medicine. Moreover, it is often assumed that an increase in female professionals in one area of the workforce has flow-on benefits to other females in the same area. But, in *Sex and Medicine*, a 1998 study of the impact of female doctors on the workforce in both Australia and the UK, Rosemary Pringle challenges such a view. Using a wide sample of female doctors, Pringle interrogated the claim that they bring a traditional feminine nurturing dimension into the male world of medicine. She notes that this perception constructs women doctors, their roles and careers in juxtaposition with their male counterparts. Certainly the pioneer women doctors in the early twentieth century were most often located in the fields of community health and women's health clinics. Like nurses of the day, they were often single middle-class women.[20] But, as Pringle points out, it is wrong to align female doctors as interested only in women's issues, or to assume that female doctors are necessarily more nurturing than male ones.

Pringle also claims that the movement of women into medicine in large numbers may, contrary to popular wisdom, have disadvantaged nursing in its struggle to gain equality in the male world of medical science. She argues that since women have been able to gain entry to medicine, it challenges the traditional notions of women being best suited to roles which require 'feminine' qualities of caring and nurturing rather than roles requiring rational thought (as if the two are mutually exclusive). Over time it has been assumed that women who went into nursing did so because they were not bright enough to enter medicine but could manage a menial role which merely required those 'natural' feminine qualities. As with most career paths, of course, the reasons for this choice are far more complex. In my case I would have had to travel to the nearest university which meant living away from home—unthinkable to my family. This was so for many other young women in the 1960s and since nursing was not then in universities, we were disadvantaged when we went on to do further studies because nursing studies were not thought of as worthy of being considered for credit or advanced standing into other studies. Pringle also highlights the tensions which have emerged between nurses and female doctors as they negotiate their roles. She records interviews with women doctors who describe difficulties they have working with female nurses: a lack of cooperation and a failure to treat them with the same deference as male doctors. Interestingly, nurses in the same study had different views, claiming that women doctors were often easier to work with, more cooperative and less arrogant and demanding than their male counterparts.

Of course, the effects of a social phenomenon such as the women's movement are difficult to measure in any definitive way because of the complex manner in which such effects interact with other social factors over time and the variables involved. It is also impossible to generalise changes to women across social, cultural and economic contexts. Certainly, the more open and inclusive modes of communication, the active consumer movements and the increasing number of educated women in the system can all be attributed, at least in part, to the influence of the women's movement.

3

THE IMPACT OF TECHNOLOGY

The scene is as clear to me today as it was then. G, an active 90-year-old woman, returned from surgery having suffered a cardiac arrest under anaesthetic. She arrived back in the ward unconscious and attached to a ventilator; her distraught children and grandchildren surrounded the bed. They asked for my reassurance since I was the nurse who had got to know their mother and grandmother, a woman who still maintained her own house and whose only dysfunction was increasing breathlessness and pain when hanging out her washing. G died on the ventilator, unable to say goodbye. The relatives of patients like G never knew that many of us questioned the decision to proceed with coronary artery bypass surgery on an elderly patient. We were silent, if unwilling, accomplices.

J, a 30-year-old strong, healthy man, was brought into the intensive care unit with an obvious brain stem head injury. When he stopped breathing, with his young pregnant wife by his side begging us to save him, the medical director of the unit hesitated only briefly before intubating him and attaching him to a ventilator. Weeks later J regained consciousness and we knew then that while the ventilator had saved his body, his brain was irreparably damaged. His young wife and child found a man they no longer knew. He certainly showed no flicker of recognition. J was and always would be in a chronic vegetative state.

Patricia had rushed home from work to prepare a special birthday dinner for her teenage son. She had felt sick for days, putting it down to a virus, so she left her husband to finish the preparation and laid down on her bed for a nap. Unable to wake her for the celebrations later that night, her husband felt helpless as he witnessed her rapid deterioration into a state of extreme delirium. Thanks to transplant technology, Patricia woke several days later to find herself with a new liver and a new life. During my career I have witnessed an enormous number of technological innovations and nursed people whose lives were changed by them. Among these are: the increasing use of 'wonder' drugs to fight once lethal infections; the use of intravenous fluid to protect trauma victims from renal failure; the ventilator and defibrillator; haemodynamic measurement by central lines rather than through rough estimations; feeding by catheters directly into the central veins; and organ donation and transplantation.

Each of these innovations comes with its many stories and memories of faces and families I can't forget. Teenagers lying between clean sheets, pink cheeks, chests raising and falling for days as tests were done to 'prove death'. Parents sitting, waiting, watching, begging me with their eyes as I washed and turned their children. Families noticing the slightest movement of limb or facial expression, waiting for a sign that it was all a big mistake. And then the final moment when the bed is wheeled out with a pink, breathing, warm child who never returns.

It is clear to most of us involved in health care now that in many cases we got it very wrong. In our enthusiasm for technological advance we forgot those who were sometimes left behind. Through the experience of caring for patients like J and G, I came to realise the profound cost of technological innovation for some patients and their families. At the same time, Patricia's rapid recovery and long-term survival are testimony to the way in which technology can have a positive affect on many lives, offering hope where once there was none. Her story is one of many 'miracles' made possible through technological innovations.

This chapter focuses on the ways in which technology has affected patients and the care they receive. It will address questions commonly asked in the era of high-tech health care: has it distanced the patient from the professional? Has the patient been lost in the lines, drains and alarms? With diagnosis increasingly dependent on tests, scans, measurements, computers and chart readings, has the environment become one where personal touch and talk has diminished, even disappeared? What are the implications for the

37

patient when the focus of the medical gaze has now shifted from the whole person to the organ, the cells in the organ, and even the DNA which makes up the cell? In short, what are the real costs of high-tech health care for patients and the way they are cared for?

RECENT TECHNOLOGICAL DEVELOPMENTS

When people think about medical technology today there is a tendency to think in terms of those technologies which are the most spectacular, such as transplantation, genetic engineering and in vitro fertilisation. Yet, although we commonly think of technology in a fairly narrow sense, any human-made invention or innovation can be regarded as technological. Accordingly, health care technology refers not only to high-tech devices such as ventilators, but also to drugs and medical and surgical procedures, and even things as basic as surgical gloves or developments in hand-washing techniques. It extends to devices which facilitate communication from patient to nurse, nurse to doctor and doctor to doctor, from the rudimentary hand-held patient call bell to the more complex telemedicine devices which transmit electro-cardiographic (ECG) traces.

I entered nursing in a time when technology in the high-tech sense of the term was in its infancy. It was in the days of mercury thermometers placed under the tongue, hand-held sphygmo-manometers, measuring the pulse by counting the beats for 60 seconds and then recording it all in three different colours. Caring for a ward of thirty patients was no mean feat. The introduction of intravenous (IV) drips into a ward was regarded as quite advanced, with only the most senior nurse being allowed to interact with the IVs. The patients attached to the IVs were identified as more complex cases requiring special observations. The ability to access the vascular system and feed fluids and blood products directly into patients' bodies was a major breakthrough for both trauma victims and surgical patients.

Later there were chambers attached to the IV lines, which not only detected air in the line but automatically measured and monitored the accuracy of the device. By then IV fluid therapy was a mainstream intervention and remains so. Today ambulance officers routinely insert IV lines before transferring a patient from an accident, and cannulas for urgent access are inserted in all patients admitted for surgery.

My memories of the first ventilator are clear because I was directly involved in nursing and saving the life of a young man with tetanus using this home-made invention. Previously this was not possible—tetanus killed. This relatively crude machine maintained his airway during enforced deep sedation. Ventilators became rapidly more sophisticated as their potential became evident. Gone now are the ventilators we had to dismantle after each patient use, to clean, scrub, soak, reassemble and test before the next patient.

Another significant breakthrough was the invention of instruments such as the ophthalmoscope and microscope, and later X-rays, ultrasounds, computerised axial tomography (CAT) and magnetic resonance imaging (MRI), all of which enabled the doctor to visualise as well as to feel and listen, adding a new dimension to the art of diagnosis. One of the major health technological innovations in the last century was the ability to obtain access to the interior of the body through catheters, scopes and radiological techniques and to insert devices which take over the function of failed or diseased parts. The cardiac pacemaker was one such innovation allowing individuals to live normal lives again after the uncertainty of living daily with life-threatening heart irregularities. Inserting catheters such as the Swan-Ganz into major arteries and veins for diagnosis or monitoring of various physical parameters, such as arterial and venous pressures and cardiac function, has become an accepted practice. Monitoring devices have become increasingly sophisticated, enabling a more accurate and immediate diagnosis and assisting in the prevention of emergencies.

Eventually, technology allowed us to save those not only with acute illnesses and injuries, but also those with terminal illnesses such as renal failure. In the renal unit where I worked, large haemodialysis machines lined the walls attached to fragile, yellowed women who looked 90 but were really 30. These were the days before renal transplantation so haemodialysis was their life line. Today, not only would transplantation be a possibility, but peritoneal dialysis is an everyday event for many individuals with failed kidneys, allowing them to lead relatively normal lives.

Innovations in pharmacological technology have complemented innovations in equipment. There has been an exponential increase in the range of drugs available to fight infections, sedate, and provide pain relief. More important, however, was a greater understanding of how drugs worked and at what doses. The discovery of the 'miracle' drugs sulpha, penicillin and streptomycin between 1930 and 1940 made a major difference in the care of those with severe infections.[1] And long surgical procedures were advanced as they relied very much on the breakthroughs in muscle relaxants which enabled patients to survive for long periods under anaesthesia. Later, the ability to keep the circulation functioning artificially outside the body meant that operations on the heart could be undertaken, from valve replacements, repair of congenital abnormalities and coronary artery bypass to heart and lung transplantation. In the case of technologies required to enable transplant surgery, improved immunosuppressant drug therapy has been one of the most important, since without such drugs patients would be unable to survive for long without rejecting their new organs. Indeed, the manufacture of the immunosuppressant drug Cyclosporin enabled liver transplantation to move from a few tentative cases to the establishment of the National Liver Transplant Unit. Transplantation of organs from one person to another symbolises for many scientists the triumph of humans over nature.

The latest technological developments centre on developing surgical interventions which reduce time spent in hospital. Keyhole surgery has provided the breakthrough here. This has enabled surgery previously done by cutting through the abdominal wall (laparotomy) to be undertaken using several small incisions through which a tiny scope can be passed. Types of surgery include hernia repair (herniorrhaphy) and gall bladder removal (cholecystectomy) but investigations, biopsies and diagnosis can also be carried out in this way, thus avoiding major surgical techniques, long anaesthetics and longer stays in hospital. Presently such surgery is under scrutiny due to some evidence of poor outcomes in a small percentage of patients. The outcomes, perhaps due to the refining of procedures, include adverse events such as damage to other internal organs due to poor vision through the scope, and extreme pain and tiredness following discharge. So despite the cost savings of 'day only' surgery, the outcomes for patients may be no better and may even be worse. This will not necessarily be clear to surgeons and hospitals, however, because the patient will be meeting the costs of staying off work longer.

IMPACT ON PATIENT CARE

Technological developments have transformed the way patient care is organised and delivered. Perhaps the most striking change has been the shift in focus from the body of the patient to the technology itself. The introduction of technological devices such as the IV drip required the attention of health care professionals, sometimes at the expense of attention to the patients. In the case of the drip, nurses had to stand beside the IV line each hour and monitor the flow in drops per minute which then allowed a calculation to be made about the amount of time it would take for the patient to receive the whole bag of fluid. My memories are of moving from bed to bed counting the IV drops per minute against my watch, and in the case of a patient receiving blood I needed to ensure that the blood was warmed through a device and that the patient was not reacting. While I always tried to remember to speak to the patient, I know that often my attention was focused on the technological detail for safety reasons.

R, a clinical nurse consultant working in both public and private hospitals today, spoke to me about the impact technology has had on her capacity to nurse as she used to a decade ago:

> Once you had six patients to manage, a few requiring technological interventions (machine or drugs). Last week I had eight patients to look after on one shift. All were acutely ill and all required technological intervention of some kind. I spent the eight hours of my shift preparing and giving medication, adjusting machinery delivering the medication, measuring the patient's physical parameters via technological devices and doing complicated wound care. I went off feeling as if I had not spent time with the person in the bed. After all, most of these patients

41

have very poor outcomes, both short and long term—actually what they want and need is to be cared for.

Interestingly, although many technological devices when first introduced were presented as time-saving, in reality the nurse has been left to ensure that, for example, the tracing leads are placed correctly on the patient, the monitor is accurate, readouts are recorded at various intervals for documentation for the doctor, and the patient is educated about the actual technology. Unlike other workplaces where it seems that the introduction of technology has cut staffing and changed the level of staff required, in health the opposite has occurred. We needed better trained staff and more of them because of the diagnostic and management possibilities and the growth of medical specialisation. While technological devices in hospitals provide more accurate data, they require skilled insertion, management and interpretation of results if the data are to be believed. Without such reassurance, the utility and safety of new technology is questionable.

As a working nurse in the 1960s, I had to learn how the new ventilators worked in addition to managing my usual workload. Intravenous therapy also meant an enormous increase in workload with the ordering and recording of fluids and management of peripheral technology such as drip counters and air bubble detectors. This is not to mention the detailed monitoring which goes on including checking orders, doses, drip rates, patient identity, additional drug therapy, individual reactions, ensuring tests are taken on time and results returned to the correct file and doctor.

In coronary care I discovered another problem. Many a patient begged me not to take him off the monitor as he was being prepared for discharge because he believed that the monitor had kept his heart beating or that the alarms alerted nurses and doctors to his abnormalities. Not only had we become dependent on the technology, so too had the patient. This was particularly true for anyone who had experienced a cardiac arrest and resuscitation. Without the monitor, how would anyone know that his heart was functioning? This dependence on the machine provided a lesson well learned for both patient and carer, and gradual weaning became an important technique with all specialist technology. I began to understand this even more during my research with patients who had undergone liver transplantation. Feeling safe was often uppermost in their stories about the surgery itself and the immediate post-operative period. This was related to the fact that their life was so dependent on machines, which in turn depended on skilled staff.

Sue spoke to me about this dependence on the machinery and the critical care unit itself where staff were meant to be highly skilled and responsive to the smallest changes in a patient. When she was on the ventilator she used to flick the pulse meter off her finger to bring the staff running to her room, just to see if she had control over her environment: 'Safety was the most important thing for me postoperatively . . . I needed to trust the people who were looking after me—after all you are there because you are unable to care for yourself.'

Another significant change brought about by increased technology in health care was the birth of widespread specialisation as we know it today. The rise in specialised machines entailed a rise in specialist units. Technology begat specialists and speciality areas, educational programs and research units and in turn they begot more sophisticated technologies. What began as one acute unit in any teaching hospital where severely ill patients were admitted, quickly spread into a plethora of highly specialised units focusing on specific body parts such as hands or kidneys, on dysfunctions such as incontinence or asthma, or on disorders which require specialised technology such as sleep apnoea or renal dialysis. Once we worked in 'Ward One', now we work in the 'Paediatric Neurology Unit'.

The impact of technology on work practices, organisation of health care, and the culture of hospitals has been enormous. I well remember the way in which specialist staff were identified as separate from the general staff in the rest of the hospital in the early days of intensive care. There was a feeling of 'them and us' pervading what had once been a culture of community throughout the hospital. Today communities seem to exist within the specialities themselves rather than throughout the organisation, except in the case of a relatively small peripheral hospital. And specialist colleges and associations have led to further fragmentation of disciplines, which in some ways has eroded any hope of a united voice in general health care matters. Vested interests understandably abide in the specialist groups rather than in the wider discipline, whether that be medicine, nursing, pharmacy or physiotherapy.

Working in specialist environments with complicated machinery we soon became specialists to survive. High-tech equipment led to the need for continual surveillance, detection and maintenance, which in turn produced a network of new industries. In the everyday routine of health care the nursing role has been most affected by such innovations. At the beginning of the twenty-first century, health care practitioners have tended to become experts in increasingly more specific areas of practice and less focused on generalist care.

THE COSTS OF HIGH-TECH HEALTH CARE

There is no doubt that technological innovations have saved and extended the lives of many patients. But, increasingly, high-tech health care has had negative effects—often unexpected—on the health and quality of life of patients. An instructive example is the introduction of a simple piece of technology such as the latex glove. Our move away from commonsense procedures, such as hand-washing, has contributed to a high incidence of infection in hospitals. Inappropriate pharmacological intervention, such as the over-prescription of antibiotics, has also contributed to the increase of 'super' infections due to the creation of new, resistant strains of bacteria. Increased pharmacological technology has also produced an increase in errors in drug dispensing. Drug 'events', as they are referred to in health care, now make up the majority of accidental or adverse incidents in hospitalised patients in the USA.[2] These drug errors occur mainly during ordering and dispensing, which appears to point to practitioner error but has been shown to be caused mainly by faulty systems. An Australian study[3] investigating the number of drug-related hospital admissions found equally concerning data. Each year at least 80 000 hospital admissions are due to medication-related problems. But while such outcomes are extremely concerning and costly, there would be little debate about the positive impact drugs have had on mortality rates and quality of life globally.

There has been a flood of litigation, particularly in the USA, relating to the health problems created by technology. A settlement trust of $4 billion in the case of Dow Corning (who manufactured silicone breast implants) was judged to be inadequate compensation for the chronic illnesses which have damaged so many women's lives. Manville, the industrial giant which manufactured asbestos—which causes mesothelioma—is bankrupt from litigation with an increasing number of cases emerging as the full impact of asbestos-related disease is revealed. Electromagnetic field radiation, which surrounds us daily through our electrical appliances, undergoes ongoing investigation for its links with cancers, as do a number of potential environmental hazards such as hydrocarbons and hydrochlorofluorocarbons (HCFCs), all part of the technological evolution. Increased litigation, ironically, has meant an increased use of technology for screening and diagnosis in the USA, with the spiral CT scan being used to diagnose relatively simple conditions such as an inflamed appendix.

Recent research has shown that even the so-called 'minimally invasive' surgery may not be so minimal in its invasiveness. There have been instances of major complications with the burden of cost shifting to the patient who may have longer off work due to pain, lethargy and infection.[4] There is also a level of concern about adverse events such as damage to other organs put down to poor visualisation of the abdominal cavity through the scope. Despite such concern, however, there is little doubt that reducing the length of time patients remain in bed after surgery has had positive outcomes in terms of the reduction of complications of bed rest which were evident in the past—complications such as chest infections and deep venous thrombosis (clotting), both requiring longer hospitalisation and further technological intervention.

Increased intervention has also meant that the first principle of immunity is breached—the first line of bodily defence, skin and mucous membrane, is broken. Parenteral feeding techniques mean that central and peripheral veins are accessed by foreign objects left in for considerable lengths of time. The upper respiratory tract is now invaded by intubation tubes and suction catheters with the potential to cause serious lung infections. Bladders are assaulted for weeks on end with catheters. All this in someone with a weakened immune system not necessarily able to resist such infection. Many patients died in the past, and still do, not because of the original trauma but because of a secondary infection. The incidence of iatrogenic disease—which is caused by medicine itself—continues to rise.

As technology transferred diagnosis from the hands of the doctor to the eyes of the technician, a new world of risk opened up alongside the potential for a more accurate diagnosis. Individual doctors who previously in their initial examination of a patient would have explored a range of diagnoses prior to settling on one, relied more heavily on technology to bypass this 'diagnosis by elimination'. We now know the risks of diagnostic testing through chance (such as false positive or negative results) or through human error (such as wrong names being entered or samples being mixed). In the early days high-tech equipment was seen as infallible. If the machines dictated a level, a measure, a parameter, it was right. No uncertainty existed. Eventually, however, we began to see that as machines broke down, as batteries failed, as patients became sicker through machine malfunctioning, high-tech equipment was as uncertain as humans— because humans made it, programmed it, organised it, used it, and interpreted the data it produced.

Another consequence of this shift in diagnostic procedures has been what some would call the 'dehumanising' of the clinical relationship. One of the most common complaints about the increased use of and reliance on technology is that it has distanced the health care professional from the patient. Specialists can now diagnose from thousands of kilometres away through the advent of telemedicine. As a result, there is often a loss of personal contact and in particular a loss of touch in the encounter between patient and doctor which may prove to be extremely negative in its effect on outcomes. There is strong empirical evidence to suggest that personal interaction plays a significant role in the healing process.

This 'dehumanising' extends to the hospital environment itself. Sue, a patient recently diagnosed with non-Hodgkins lymphoma who had to undergo a CAT scan, describes her experience of the hospital environment this way: 'I think the main problem is at the entrance. Hospitals are supposed to be care facilities but what greets you is information technology: faxes, computers, flashing lights and paging systems. The most human element about the hospital was the lady giving out tea and coffee.' In addition, many patients are nursed in environments which are not at all therapeutic. Brightly lit units and extremely sensitive alarms provide a continuous cacophony of sound, day and night, along with call bells, telephones and emergency alerts producing a background filled with white noise. We introduce patients whose bodies have failed, who are sedated and frightened, and who are continuously being monitored and invaded into this environment.

R, recently diagnosed with mesothelioma, spoke to me of the anger she felt about the offhand way she had been treated in two very high-tech areas of a large teaching hospital:

> It was two days of tests in the Nuclear Medicine department and he [the head of department] told us that we would know at the end of that time if I would respond to the treatment. It was pretty important to me! I came in after two days to be told that he had flown to Paris and hadn't left instructions. My anger was that it was my body and somebody was going to know things and they were not permitted to tell me about it. He [the specialist] had left nothing in progress to inform me and to this day I have never heard from him. I waited one month and then worked through another specialist. The hardest part was not that I couldn't have the treatment, I could handle that, but that somebody treated me as if I was of no importance to him— maybe because I was of no further use . . . I was treated as a non-person during that time in the Nuclear Medicine department and in Radiology. I've never been treated like that—maybe it was just the personnel—I wasn't used to that. I had a feeling that it was a different mentality, as if you didn't have any rights.

While it makes no sense to generalise from one story, there is no doubt that technology sometimes intervenes to save lives without paying attention to the quality of the life we leave behind. Take, for example, A, head of a large corporation. He understood the meaning of control, both being in and keeping control. He had a major heart attack which destroyed a large part of his cardiac muscle. To save his life we inserted an assistive device into his aorta to take much of the cardiac workload and allow his heart to rest. This was the era of the intra-aortic balloon pump which had been hailed as the future of cardiology. It was still to be evaluated. I continued to nurse him. His family were bewildered, looking to me for answers as to how this huge and powerful man could have been reduced to the frail body in the bed attached to lines into every orifice, unable to sit up or eat. After some time we attempted to remove the device and test his heart's capacity. Each time we were forced to reinsert it. We kept him alive through an artificial device and drugs as his family struggled to keep their hopes alive. One day he demanded to know why I hadn't let him die, why had I subjected him to this humiliation as I assisted in the most intimate aspects of his daily living? He was very angry. And of course I wondered about the same thing, but being young and relatively inexperienced I had no answers, and could only offer platitudes about looking forward, not giving in and considering his family. My answers today would have been entirely different—more honest in terms of his future and how he might be involved in decisions about any future intervention. One day we had no choice but to remove the device. I remember him being wheeled out of the intensive care unit to a general cardiology ward, still struggling to breathe or speak. He knew his fate.

In the unit his survival was hailed as a success. The intensive care statistics recorded him as a 'save'. As I said my goodbyes I wondered how he and his family would adjust to the fact that he was now a cardiac invalid for the rest of his life. His wife had already spoken with me of her fears about looking for a job. She had always stayed at home. He was the breadwinner. Once more I wondered about my part in saving a patient at the cost of his quality of life. In the case of A, however, I didn't have to wonder for long. After all the intervention he had a final heart attack and died before being discharged.

WHERE TO FROM HERE?

Too often debates about technology either simplistically demonise or valorise technological advancements in medicine uncritically. In reality, the impact of technology on health care has neither created all our problems nor solved them. Undoubtedly, new technology has saved lives which previously could not have been saved. Just as surely, it has created a new set of problems. Successful organ transplantation techniques were made possible by pharmacological discoveries which decreased rejection rates. As a result of this pharmacological intervention, however, patients developed diseases such as lymphoma caused by long-term immunosuppression. Long distance diagnosis has collapsed the distance of people in remote areas from health care services but at the same time it may distance the practitioner from the patient.

Not only are we seeing an increased number of drug resistant infections and adverse events through medical intervention, we are grappling with major ethical problems thrown up by an increasingly technologised health care system. Issues relate to equity and access to health care, such as what research and development should be funded, which expensive equipment should be situated where, or whose lives should be saved and who we should allow to die.

Governments are increasingly shifting the burden of responsibility onto the public both in terms of cost and in terms of the care itself. Yet, although ordinary people are more implicated in the institution of health care than ever before, public debate concerning which medical innovations are and are not acceptable or desirable, and therefore which innovations should be funded, is extremely limited.

There has been a preoccupation in popular debates in recent times with the ethics of biotechnology. There is constant speculation, for example, about the way in which techniques such as cloning will alter the shape of our existence. As a recent report from the NSW Innovation Council, *Biotechnology in NSW: Opportunities and Challenges*, puts it:

> Biotechnology is one of the two great generic technologies of our times which, with information technology, is profoundly altering our society . . . The impact of biotechnology is just starting to be felt. The technology is so powerful and developing at such a speed that it is difficult even to predict how it will change our lives in the next century.[5]

What needs much more urgent attention in public debate, however, is the question of the appropriate uses of medical intervention today. Innovations such as life maintenance machines, organ transplantation and genetic manipulation do not come cheaply, either in terms of money or of people's lives. They require the shift of money previously allocated to other areas, which results in funding inequities across the various sectors of health care. Surely the public funding already allocated to health should be directed to the major health problems facing people today, those health problems which cause most patients to seek medical care? The ten most frequently managed problems are hypertension, upper respiratory tract infection, immunisation, bronchitis, depression, asthma, back complaints, diabetes, high cholesterol, and osteoarthritis,[6] none of which would necessarily benefit from high-tech intervention and all of which can be mainly managed by general practitioners. Yet the bulk of the state health budget goes to hospitals and acute interventions, and not to the chronic illness side of health care. Meanwhile, general practitioners are funded by the federal government and, because of funding mechanisms, are restricted in the time they can afford to spend with each patient. Patients suffering from any one of these ten problems need time with a practitioner who can advise them about the best way to manage their disease and minimise its effects on their life. The allocation of funding and other resources needs extensive questioning when it comes to meeting the health needs of the majority in our society.

Technological innovation has certainly added considerably to the cost of health care, not just because of the innovation itself but because it adds yet another level of practitioner and practice to a crowded field. The paradox of high-tech innovation is that at the same time that we are prepared to fund high-tech 'miracle' interventions we are told there is insufficient funding for very basic health care which could improve the primary health of disadvantaged groups in the community.

With every new technological breakthrough, including new drugs, specialists emerge, educational courses are launched, research centres are funded. As institutions and practices become entrenched, so do investments in them. High-tech interventionist practices are taken for granted, both within the health care system and outside by patients whose expectations are inevitably raised. As new drugs are developed and new procedures become available, patients demand the latest interventions and practitioners ensure they are delivered. But with this comes the associated costs to individuals and to the health care system, costs which the public either are ignorant of or choose, often for very good reasons, to ignore. Another problem with innovations is that many practices are introduced without evaluation and remain without evidence of their effectiveness in terms of patient outcomes.

Once large organ transplantation became possible it quickly became a standard option on the medical treatment list. While centres were set up in an experimental capacity, they very rapidly became established centres supported by ongoing public funding. Long-term outcomes, of course, may not be positive but are rarely assessed once an individual becomes a successful statistic—a 'survivor'[7]—measured by the fact that they were discharged from hospital. Is the enormous cost of such high-tech intervention—including the financial outlay, the potential negative long-term outcomes, as well as the cost of not putting our resources elsewhere—one that the public would be willing to pay if they were better informed about the bigger picture of health care? Any debates that are conducted about these issues are held behind closed doors.

In spite of the lack of public debate, there is evidence that the public is not entirely satisfied with what high-tech scientific medicine has to offer them. Technological innovations have increased but so too has the interest in alternative therapies. One explanation of this trend could be that people are seeking alternatives to the technological model of health care which 'dehumanises' the patient and focuses on illness rather than health and well-being. It is possible that rather than seen as antagonistic to conventional medicine, alternative therapies will come to complement it by fulfilling patients' needs for being cared for holistically while at the same time having access to high-tech intervention in acute circumstances.

The move away from generalist expertise has left patients wanting a good clinician who is able to look at them as a whole person and not just as a compilation of parts. Patients complain that doctors tend to focus on one or two aspects of their health problem rather than exercising lateral thinking and using good clinical judgement. General practitioners are criticised for relying on high-tech solutions such as drugs and referrals to specialists.

Even in nursing, generic practitioners are much needed today in the acute system where efficiency requires that nurses move between speciality areas according to need. This is difficult for the nurse who has worked in one particular speciality for several years. Of course, generalists are found in the remote and some rural areas of Australia because of the lack of practitioners in these areas. There is the added problem of the lack of specialist facilities, often due to the lack of a sufficient population to support them.

Patients, it seems, have conflicting feelings about technological intervention. On the one hand they demand it and even become dependent on it, but on the other there is widespread condemnation of the technological age and its 'dehumanising' effects. But there is also an added factor—safety. While patients in the 1960s entered hospital for safety reasons they are now discharged or leave for the same reasons. Hospitals are dangerous, a fact recognised at a national level through the setting up of a National Expert Advisory Group on Safety and Quality in Australian Health Care.[8] This points to some recognition that there needs to be a re-evaluation of the unbridled use of technology in health care.

The impact of technology within the area of health has been enormous. It has altered the way in which we think about health, illness, death and life. It has demanded new disciplines, disciplinarians, practices and practitioners and altered the distribution of funding in a way which has had long-term implications for certain groups in our society. It has raised our expectations and our sense of where we stand in the scheme of things. Some are all-powerful, some have lost power. Mortal infections have been cured with antibiotics, we can prevent disease through vaccination, and now not only do we remove diseased parts, we replace them. As a result, social expectations have increased and in turn have further driven the push for high-tech health care solutions. But such solutions may only be short term since enabling people to live longer lives means leaving them exposed to illnesses they would not have encountered had their lives been shorter. When women died in childbirth, they were not left to face breast and uterine cancer, osteoarthritis, osteoporosis and dementia. When men died of heart attacks at a younger age and in larger numbers than is presently so, they were not left to face cancer of the prostate and dementia.

As a result, health problems are becoming increasingly more complex and the range of demands on the health care system more competitive and costly, leading to health being reconceptualised as a business.

4

THE COMMODIFICATION OF
HEALTH CARE

S spoke to me of her recent experience with her small son who was sick and in need of immediate attention. She rushed to the nearest emergency department because she was increasingly worried about his condition.

> He was getting sicker and I know how quickly children can deteriorate. I waited and waited at the emergency department worried all the time, but after 4 hours I gave up and went home. I assumed that we were not seen as an emergency—actually nobody came and told me anything but I just gave up.

S's story is one of many. As I write this book there is intense media focus on the apparent 'crisis' in our public hospitals. Television news and current affairs programs constantly run dramatic television interviews with distressed families forced to wait hours in emergency departments. And examples of the 'breakdown' of the health care system often make front page news in the nation's daily press:

Hospital unable to cope as it bleeds from fiscal cuts!!![1]
For the past four years Prince of Wales Hospital has overrun its budget by about $9 million . . . The result has been 250 beds closed, 270 staff lost and doctors unable to give their patients the care they think they deserve. According to the clinical director of surgery Dr Robert Farnsworth, patients are sent home before they are well enough. 'We are now pushing patients out of the hospital because there are not the beds to keep them in', he said.

Sydney's Sickest Hospital![2]

At Westmead Hospital, patients with bowel cancer must wait four to six weeks for surgery while those with breast cancer face delays of about a month, medical staff have revealed. 'This place is on a knife edge', Professor Kefford [chairman of the division of medicine] said. 'Sometimes I drive home in the evening biting my fingernails literally and think, "God I hope there isn't a disaster".'

Hospital emergency; it's getting worse . . . people can't take the pressure any more[3]

Ambulance officers yesterday joined the outcry over Sydney's funding crisis saying they were forced to spend hours in emergency departments waiting for patients to be transferred from trolleys to beds.

There is no denying that hospitals and, in particular, emergency departments are extraordinarily busy and often have patients waiting to be seen, waiting for tests, waiting for decisions, waiting to be taken home by ambulance, waiting for medication, waiting for a dressing, waiting for the specialist. But the reasons for this are perhaps not as clear as some media reports suggest. The cause of these problems in our current system is the result of budget cuts. What this analysis fails to recognise though is that budget restrictions are only one aspect of the much more complex phenomenon of what we might call the 'commodification' of health care.

Increasingly, the health care system has been subject to economic pressures which have resulted in a variety of changes to the organisation of the health care system and, therefore, in the delivery of health services. We have seen bed cuts in public hospitals, an increase in cheaper but less qualified nursing staff, new models of health service delivery, a decrease in the length of stay in hospital, particularly for surgical patients, and the standardisation of practices through benchmarking and costing of individual and hospital practices. While undoubtedly some of these changes have been well overdue, others have been condemned by professional groups who see some government implemented changes as undermining the health professional's clinical judgements about what is best for each patient. This chapter will look at some of the complexities of this so-called drive to commodification in health care, the ways in which it has shaped the current system, and the advantages and disadvantages of the changes associated with it for patient care.

THE POLITICS OF HEALTH CARE

The right of all Australians to access health care as they need it is a value that most people, indeed virtually all of us, would uphold. The sometimes vast differences between individuals and groups on the matter of health care arise over the detail of this ideal, specifically, how it should be delivered, who should ensure its maintenance and quality, and how to organise such a system. And all of these are in turn tied to the general problem of funding.

Sydney Sax, Chairman of the National Hospitals and Health Services Commission in 1973, pointed to two principal groups as the major players in the determination of the economics of health care, and in particular the evolution of national health insurance, in Australia: politicians and doctors.[4]

Of course, the government of the day, as holder of the public purse, has the ultimate say over how funds are spent. Palmer and Short claim that in Australia health has been a major political issue in every federal election since 1969 and, as such, funding decisions have been consistently informed by the ideological beliefs of the political force in power.[5] Labor Prime Minister Chifley in 1943 declared his commitment to a comprehensive national welfare scheme which included health services. But Earl Page, Minister for Health (and also a founding fellow of the Royal Australasian College of Surgeons) in the Liberal–Country Party government in 1949, expressed his party's ideological opposition to such a system: 'The great danger in any government aided health scheme is the tendency to develop a psychology of dependency and diminished personal and community responsibility.'[6] Judgements about who were the 'deserving' underpinned Liberal policies, while Labor's position was traditionally more one of ensuring protection for all, thus their push for a national health insurance and other welfare supports.

In 1949 the Labor government fell from power and some would say this was largely because they had placed a comprehensive *National Health Act* on the statute books. The elected Liberal government abandoned this Act in favour of a privately funded contributory scheme devised in consultation with the British Medical Association (BMA). At this time doctors in Australia were yet to form their own association and were members of the BMA. This scheme was described as 'private practice publicly supported' since it meant that medical practitioners were supported by government funding as well as being privately funded by patients in many cases.[7] This new scheme was supported by growth in private insurance companies such as the Medical Benefits Fund (MBF), sponsored by the medical professions, and the Hospital Contribution Funds (HCF), controlled by public hospitals, both of which were set up in the same year.

Because this new health scheme left many groups without access to health services, the Liberal government introduced the Pensioner Medical Service which covered those receiving pensions such as the aged, the disabled and the widowed. Over time this service underwent many changes, leading to a means test being applied to appease many doctors who felt somewhat exploited by being providers at concessional rates to people they believed had the means to pay.

In 1969 the Nimmo Committee was set up by the Liberal government to answer Labor's questions on medical and hospital costs. This led to recommendations about a standard schedule of medical fees which, because of the contentious nature of such a recommendation, led to a split in the, by then, Australian Medical Association (AMA). A small group broke away to form the General Practitioners' Society but the major group of doctors accepted the arrangement with limitations, namely that this would not be a definitive schedule of fees but would merely provide information about a range of fees ultimately determined by the individual doctor. This became enshrined in the *Health Benefits Act* of 1970.

Perhaps the most radical reforms relating to the funding and provision of public health were initiated after the Whitlam Labor government came to power in 1972. These reforms were informed by Whitlam's visionary approach but it must be said that the climate was also right due to increasingly informed consumers discontented with the system as it was. Whitlam conceived of health care in the broadest possible terms, much more widely than simply as an issue of hospital intervention. The Whitlam government's policies reflected a recognition of the many elements which impact on the health of individuals and families, including housing, education, family support, nutrition and employment. These elements had been well documented but, by and large, ignored by previous governments, save for the occasional attempt at the integration of services. In contrast, The Hospitals and Health Commission established by the Whitlam government was charged with establishing a network of integrated services, with primary care as the cornerstone.

In 1974, after fierce opposition from the AMA, who viewed 'socialised' medicine as a retrograde step, Medibank, a universal health insurance scheme, was established in Australia. Doctors providing care for patients in public hospitals were paid as salaried staff or visiting medical officers (VMOs) where previously there had been an honorary system. For non-hospital consultations doctors could either bulk-bill patients and then bill Medibank for the scheduled fee, or charge the patient up-front. The patient then needed to make a claim on Medibank. This rather complex system was set up to overcome the earlier concerns by the medical profession when they challenged the *Pharmaceutical Benefits Act* of 1947 which had attempted to set a schedule of fees. As highly educated professionals, doctors believed that they were better able to determine the value of a service. They were also concerned that bureaucratic intervention undermined the integrity of their relationship with the patient.

Following the dismissal of the Whitlam Labor government in 1975, Liberal Prime Minister Malcolm Fraser aimed for social equity via competition rather than regulation. Medibank II emerged in an effort to reinstate private health insurance and win the support of the AMA, but a series of amendments in 1978 and 1979 changed the system of full reimbursement to a repayment up to the scheduled fee of all fee charges in excess of $20.[8]

Tension between the federal and state governments in terms of funding different sections of health was an ongoing problem and remains so. One of the main changes under the Fraser government was the removal of state grants tied to specific projects and their replacement with block grants, thus shifting the responsibility for resource allocation to the states. This had severe funding disadvantages for programs such as the Community Health Program set up under the Whitlam regime to ensure a coordinated community health care approach integrating services between federal and state funding and institutions and the community. Hawke's Labor government came to power in 1983 and immediately set about re-establishing centralised control over health funding. Medibank was renamed Medicare and was financed through a progressive tax levy collected by the federal government. This remains the case at the time of writing, although the taxed percentage has risen from 1 per cent to between 1.5 and 2.5 per cent, depending on the taxpayer's gross salary.

Although decisions about the funding of health care are ultimately in the hands of the government of the day, doctors, as it should now be clear, have continued to exert a powerful influence over how the health care system is organised and particularly how funds are distributed. Doctors lobbied for the defeat of the national health insurance scheme proposed by the 1948 Labor government, for example. When the Liberal Party came to power, the medical profession had an ally of sorts in Earl Page, the Minister for Health. His understanding of the culture of medicine and his credibility with the then BMA, of which he was a member, meant that he was sympathetic to the agenda of the profession. His revised version of the national health insurance scheme was forged out of an agreement between the government and the BMA.

The medical profession has had considerable success in blocking changes to legislation and funding models whenever it appeared that they might lose their independence from government control.[9] In 1943 the then Labor government legislated for a Pharmaceutical Benefits Scheme (PBS) similar to the one we now have in place, but the BMA refused to put it into practice.[10] When the Chifley Labor government legislated a second *Pharmaceutical Benefits Act* in 1947, which made it a punishable offence to prescribe on anything but a government form, the BMA challenged this in court on the grounds that it constituted civil conscription and they won the day. Thus it was that doctors and dentists were freed from the compulsion to 'engage in a particular occupation, perform particular work or perform work in a particular way'.[11]

Today the AMA remains the most politically powerful group within health. And while the medical profession, by asserting the importance of their independent status in the system,[12] have come into conflict with governments on the issue of health care funding in an age of economic rationalism, this has not yet translated into any real erosion of their influence. For example, private medical specialists remain independent in terms of charges, despite the considerable economic pressure this puts on both the public and the private health systems.

THE IMPACT ON HEALTH CARE DELIVERY

In Australia the demand for health care has increased annually (if the percentage of funds allocated to health in federal and state budgets is a valid indicator); there has been a 50 per cent increase from 1960 to 1990.[13] A common government response to rising costs has been to cut funding and therefore resources—in particular cutting staff, closing beds and reducing patients' length of stay. These changes have had a profound effect on the way in which health care professionals deliver their care and the type of care available.

Recently the Independent Pricing and Regulatory Tribunal stated that 70 per cent of the increased costs in the NSW public health system were due to labour and oncosts.[14] Staffing is, therefore, naturally seen as a target for economic rationalising by those who deal with budgets rather than patients. Since the nursing workforce is the largest group in the system and appears simply as a cost in the budget, cuts to nursing can amount to considerable savings in straight dollar terms, however, in terms of quality of care the cost is high. Sicker patients, requiring more intense nursing and medical care, along with other factors, certainly contribute to an increase in workload in our contemporary hospitals. The additional factors include: population growth, rising community expectations, changes in clinical practice, expanded range of service provision, growth in non-invasive surgical procedures, growing capacity to treat, advances in technology, attempts to meet unmet need, and an awareness of legal liability which translates into defensive medicine and even defensive nursing.[15]

As well as cutting staff, another rationalisation strategy is to reduce bed numbers. Bed cuts have also meant that some public patients wait for surgery, despite special funding provided to reduce waiting lists. Such reductions have been blamed for the number of patients waiting in emergency departments for admission (termed 'access block'), although this is certainly not the only or the main cause. M, a clinical nurse consultant who has been in the system for thirty years, reflects on the current state of the system for nursing practice:

> The workload for nurses has become unsafe in many ways. The ratio of patients per nurse has increased at the same time as patients are sicker, all requiring technological interventions which become the responsibility of the nurse. Thus they require increased observation and management. There is no down time like there used to be when some of your patients were able to partially care for themselves as they were recovering. Now they are discharged before that time so all patients are in the acute phase. The frustration in not being able to provide appropriate care gets to you in the end. That is why so many expert nurses leave the system . . . But the health care system and patient care are suffering because of the lack of nursing expertise.

Reduction in the length of stay in hospital has been another major economic management strategy over the past five years nationally and internationally. Many surgical patients stay in hospital for only half the time of their counterparts of only two years ago. For many who have no support in the community, early discharge poses its own difficulties. In the wake of drastically reduced hospital stays we need other models of care to ensure that patients' needs are still met in the community after discharge. In many cases families and friends have now taken up the care and cost of education and support which were once done by the hospital. This shift of costs to the community has also occurred with the aged and the mentally and physically disabled, although there is some evidence that care of the acutely mentally ill is under review as a federal priority.

B, who has been involved in numerous consumer groups and is therefore privy to many stories about accessing health care, believes that decisions are already being made about who to treat and who not to treat according to age and ability to pay. Her own recent experience reinforced this:

> I turned up at emergency with a broken wrist . . . Colley's fracture . . . and the questions I was asked were: 'How old are you and what's your occupation?' The fact that I was 69 and retired from full time work meant that my hand was not as important and my arm was merely put into a plaster, although later it required surgery.

Our present system of federal and state funding also adds to the complexities of service delivery with the federal government mainly funding general practitioners, aged care and community care, and state funding being shared across health services for hospitals and linked services. This makes it more difficult to co-ordinate care across the continuum of the health system because of cost shifting between the sectors. Many patients present to an emergency department which is state funded rather than going to a general practitioner because it offers a 'one stop shop' in terms of diagnosis, investigation and treatment without an up-front fee.

Meanwhile, general practitioners have become burdened as a result of changes in hospital practices with cost shifting the opposite way. They now handle many of the problems resulting from early discharge and while they have support mechanisms in the city, in rural and remote areas, where services have been reduced, there are fewer doctors. Indeed, many communities rely on nurses for all their health care needs, supplemented by the occasional medical clinic.

As far as access to and equity of service delivery are concerned, specialisation has particularly affected small communities who are unable to compete for resources or staff against large city teaching hospitals with highly specialised staff. Thus centres and individuals lose out to others in terms of resources, both technical and human. Many staff will only be attracted to institutions that have the latest technological capabilities, in turn offering the opportunity to undertake research and education with other specialists. And it is difficult to argue that a small hospital with limited staffing is the best place for specialised medical interventions to take place.

This lack of access and equity for patients is particularly so for patients in rural and remote areas or communities which are less attractive in terms of financial incentives, in particular Aboriginal communities. Rationalisation of services has meant that small hospitals have been downsized, with expensive technology and services centralised. We now have boutique hospitals which offer specialised services. Many services, which were previously delivered in hospital, have been moved to the home and are carried out by the patient, family or friends supported by a specialist nurse. The era of the travelling patient has introduced severe financial implications for those forced to come to large city centres for radiotherapy or regular consultation, with the cost of accommodation compounding the issue.

THE IMPACT ON PATIENTS

Of course, the multiple changes in how health care is organised in both urban and rural areas have had an effect on the patient's experience of care. There is a feeling prevailing among patients that individualised care is disappearing. This may very well be so. With the considerable reduction in a patient's time in hospital there is certainly less time to develop relationships with nurses or doctors, a factor magnified by the increased reliance on casual nursing staff and increased emphasis on technology. D's comments reflect her perception that individualised care has disappeared: 'I vomited once and no-one came. You are at their mercy [the nurses], you don't want to have to fight for your rights.' Another patient told me of her first trip to the shower after surgery: 'The nurse told me to make my way to the shower . . . I showered and waited and waited. In desperation I rang the red emergency button . . . so I struggled naked and wet to open the door.' Sometimes patients attempted to explain these delays. A common refrain was, 'The nurses are overworked and there are severe staff shortages'.

It seems likely, however, that the idea that we have lost attentive, personalised care is not completely based in reality. I have vivid memories of the depersonalised way in which we were taught to care for patients decades ago. As nurses we did tasks *to* patients rather than caring *for* the total needs of each patient. We woke patients out of their sleep so that all the washes could get done before the doctors did their rounds that day, for example.

But whether care has become more depersonalised or not, it remains the case that patients, in light of the sense of vulnerability which surrounds illness, need to be able to trust the professionals and the system, and this does not appear currently to be the case. It appears that one of the most significant factors in patients feeling that they are being neglected is the increased business of health care practitioners. General practitioners and hospital staff are under increasing pressure to push through patients. At the same time, patients complain about endless waiting.

While consumers are willing to challenge the system when they are well, many have spoken to me of how quickly they take on the passive patient role when sick. This resignation to less individualised care seems incongruent in light of the apparent rise in consumer political power, perhaps pointing to the physical and emotional vulnerability of the very ill, who do not have the physical and emotional resources to question the care or the carer.

QUESTIONING THE 'HEALTH AS COMMODITY' MODEL

The one thing all sides appear to agree on is that the health care system, no matter what form it takes, should always adhere to the fundamental ideal of equity and access for all. Given that this has obviously not been achieved in our current system, what changes need to be effected so that our future health care system ensures such an ideal?

One approach to this question has been to take issue with the health as commodity model itself. As Mark Cormack, the National Director of the Australian Healthcare Association, stated recently when calling for a national inquiry into the health care system:

> The current debate raging in the media is narrow, divisive, blame oriented and fails to recognise the common problem that we

share . . . We continue to see disadvantaged groups such as Aborigines, rural communities, the elderly and those on low incomes suffering a lower level of general health. At the same time access to state government programs such as public hospital care, community health, mental health, drug and alcohol and preventive health programs is strained to levels the community find difficult to understand.[16]

John Ralston Saul points out that accessibility to free health care is a thing of the past at the very time when it is needed more than ever before. As he says:

Life expectancy in Central Africa is 43 and dropping, one third of the children in the world are undernourished, and 30 per cent of the workforce are unemployed . . . Relying on governments of the day to fix such major social inequities seems an impossible dream in a society where every sector and institution is seen as a marketplace; an opportunity to sell a product at the greatest profit possible. This means eliminating jobs, not creating them.[17]

Saul's position is challenged by Steven Schwartz, Vice Chancellor of Murdoch University, who believes instead that Australia needs to develop 'an open, informed and competitive health market in which patients have choices and are free to act responsibly'.[18] Schwartz takes the position that health is an industry because it has an effect on a nation's economy just as any industry does; thus it should be left to the same market forces which other businesses or commodities are left to. There is certainly clear evidence now that this is already so. Where services are offered, more patients access them. Production in health certainly increases consumption. Research has linked a number of interventions such as caesarean section (CS) with whether a woman was privately insured, rather than with need. In 1996 there was an overall 1.5 per cent increase in CS in Australia but in private patients the increase was closer to 4 per cent.[19] But is this what we want and whose interests does it serve? It certainly points to inequities in terms of choice, which is the main anomaly in Schwartz's position. Freedom to choose is of course dependent on socio-economic position.

Schwartz also challenges the view that health is sacred because of its necessity for life, using food as an example of another life necessity but one which attracts no levy such as health does through Medicare. In moving health to a competitive marketplace in which restrictions on the numbers of practitioners are removed and consumers are rewarded for seeking medical attention only when absolutely necessary, he believes that not only will costs be cut but that quality will be improved. These are interesting proposals given that we have some evidence that increasing the numbers of medical practitioners leads to increased servicing.[20]

Dr Keith Suter, a social commentator and consultant to the Australian Institute of Health and Welfare, criticises the contemporary reliance on markets to predict the future.[21] He calls for strategies that integrate health and wellness into other political agendas such as education and training. Jim Hyde, in his address to a WHO SID-Rockefeller Seminar in Geneva (which was repeated in his paper at the Health Services Association conference in July 1999), also reinforced the need to look more widely for determinants of health if we are to rethink equity and health, to go outside the medical framing up of health and illness to social and economic determinants.[22]

When this wider view is taken, real changes in the health of communities are possible and have been demonstrated through various community development projects which have actively engaged the local communities. Many nurses working in the rural and remote areas of health know this only too well and have become intimately involved in working with community groups to ensure a variety of initiatives which affect the health of the community. In Tambar Springs, for example, Julie, a clinical nurse consultant, has begun an opportunity shop to ensure that families have access to adequate clothing. And in Nundle, Sue, a community nurse, holds education programs in the hotel bar to educate men about health issues such as prostate cancer.

But Hyde warns of 'the pitfalls that those working in partnerships can face, from resistance and tradition and special interest groups to direct opposition from elites that hold power which may be threatened from a broader diffusion of knowledge and control'.[23] Such resistance is evident today as the Federal Minister for Health in Australia attempts to address the cost of health care through the capping of medical fees. The move has been branded as threatening the professional relationship of doctors and patients and the independence of doctors.

While there is definitely an argument on the grounds of what a doctor is worth and how well service can be delivered if fees are predetermined, it is unclear how the capping of fees alters either the professional relationship or the independence of a doctor in making clinical decisions. Of course, arguments concerning issues of equity and affordability would also be refreshing in such a debate since health care is only influential in outcomes if it gets to those who most require it. And we now have clear evidence of the links between indicators of social capital and mortality rates.[24] Social capital indicators include income inequalities, social trust and group membership, all those things which contribute to the networks, friendships and norms so essential to communities if they are to be sustainable and successful leading to improved health status in the community itself.

WHERE TO NOW?

In many ways the shift from a welfare state to a market state is now almost complete, even in Australia where we have so far managed to hold onto a proportion of publicly funded health and welfare sectors. There is a fraying around the edges of our public systems with an increasing number of private hospitals entering the health care sector and policies developed by the federal government specifically targeted at raising the number of those privately insured in an attempt to shift costs.

While there has been some attempt to contain costs through the usual marketplace strategies, such as outsourcing, case mix funding and increased competition, there has been little attempt to address the major causes of our increasing health care costs. These can be summarised as the proliferation of technology, the increasing amount of surgical intervention (see Chapter 3) and the uncapped nature of private specialist fees.

Of course there is no denying that the world we are in today is vastly different from that of twenty years ago or even that of ten years ago, and, as such, it demands different solutions. But for

solutions to be found there needs to be a recognition of this difference. For example, programs such as Early Discharge and Hospital in the Home are increasing as our frail elderly population is
growing, yet in our society an increasing number of people are
living alone. Where are the carers for these people? All these shifts
appear to be based on the assumption that there is somebody at
home to pick up the care and the costs which governments are
abandoning. Society and health care have lost much of their
unpaid and undervalued help, but governments seem not to
recognise this fact.

As we enter the twenty-first century we are seeing the long-
term problems of a system which has been fiddled with at every
change of government since 1953 when health insurance was first
introduced,[25] rather than rethought in light of the changing
culture. No wonder there is a feeling of chaos and uncertainty,
and no wonder the solution so frequently offered is merely to
increase the budget. The more worrying thing in all this is the
proposal by several politicians and some doctors that this money
should come from consumers. Dr Dana Wainwright, a candidate
for the presidency of the AMA in 1999, claimed that 'For too
long, patients who can afford to pay have not paid enough'. This
popular view of what is wrong was rejected by Professor Stephen
Leeder several days later. As he said: 'Medicare is a universal health
insurance system paid for by us all and that covers everyone, rich
and poor. The rich contribute much more to it because of their
taxes and higher levies. They should be able to use Medicare
when they need it.'[26]

The Federal Minister for Health, Dr Michael Wooldridge,
claims to be determined to 'reform' the system but at this stage
there is only limited evidence that he has been able to do so.[27]
While he is reformist in his approach in terms of changing the
focus from illness to health, his argument once again centres on
economic rather than social factors. Predictions are that health
care costs will double within the next twenty-five years, a fright-
ening matter for any politician in our present world where
rewards are only for those who come in on budget.

But where is the argument for what percentage of gross
domestic product is the ideal to be spent on health? And who
decides this? For example, as far as Aboriginal health is concerned

we may need to double our spending for a period in order to right past inequities; we need to provide education of indigenous health workers, culturally appropriate facilities and treatments, and adequate housing and sanitation. This is not to argue that budgets are to be ignored, but it is to argue for more equitable use of funding. Not for more to be spent but for what we have to be spent more wisely. Presently a small percentage of our society has access to the latest technology and miracle surgery, while a large percentage has inadequate access to even the most basic of care.

Hard decisions are required for moving funds from one sector to ensure the beginning of equity across sectors. Meanwhile, we need to ensure that those things which are working are protected. The benefits of Medicare are clear when compared on a number of criteria to the free enterprise system of the USA, where the level of care is determined by large private insurance enterprises whose major goal is profit. American newspapers are full of horror stories of people having to drive hundreds of kilometres with a very sick child to reach the hospital which the managed care company has approved as one of the centres they can access if they want a rebate.[28] Only the very poor are covered through a government assistance scheme.

Despite the increasing cost of technology, our health expenditure as a percentage of gross domestic product runs around 8.2 per cent while the North American percentage has blown out to around 14 per cent. In terms of access to health care, the lack of a publicly funded system (except for the poverty stricken) has left 40 million Americans uninsured and the system itself controlled by private insurance companies whose central aim is profit before high quality patient care.

Australians also have a higher than average life expectancy in relation to health care expenditure when compared with other developed countries, although it must be pointed out that this is not so for our indigenous groups whose life expectancy is only half that of the rest of our population. Such inequity continues to be reflected across society in terms of unequal access to the same standard of care. While this is apparent in overt ways, such as in the two-tiered system of public or private accommodation or even access to facilities, it is also expressed covertly in terms of waiting times or length of consultations.

We already know that the twenty-first century will bring with it an increasing number of people who require management outside the acute-oriented system—people already disadvantaged in terms of funding distribution but who make up large sectors of our communities and whose basic health needs are not being met while others receive miracle cures. We will have an increasingly ageing population, an increasing number of people living with chronic conditions, increasing socially produced problems such as depression and drug dependence, and most likely a larger population of people living below the poverty line. The most urgent problem facing the current health care system, then, is ensuring that these people (like all others in our community) will have access to the highest quality care at all times.

As the Commonwealth's share of health costs rose (from 25 per cent in the period between 1945–46 to 55 per cent by 1969–70) obvious questions were raised concerning the benefit of such financial outlay in terms of the nation's health status. And given the evidence that health status is mainly determined by factors such as genetics, environment, lifestyle and socioeconomic conditions, it is questionable whether our health care system, structured as it is around acute intervention, has any impact on health status—although it may on illness status. After all, our hospitals treat people who are already diseased. The areas which have shown improvements through acute intervention have been those where lives have been saved through procedures such as coronary artery bypass and transplantation. Infant mortality, while an indicator of a nation's health status, is not solely linked to medical intervention but also to improved education, better birth control and therefore fewer at-risk pregnancies, and better antenatal care, to name but a few factors. Where these are absent, infant mortality rates remain high.

Despite all the indicators alerting us to anomalies in the system, decisions about funding remain mainly focused on hospitals—and these are very different today from those of the early 1980s and vastly different from those of the 1960s. Ironically, such difference is the result of medicine's success in terms of curing previously fatal diseases and higher survival rates through increasingly sophisticated technologies.[29] The proliferation of stories about 'miracle' cures naturally increases the public's expectations and the costs. B, who works as a clinical nurse consultant in critical care areas, observes:

> Everyone expects to have the latest test and surgery now. They come into hospital knowing what investigations and drugs are the latest and they expect them. Relatives actually demand them. Many have written information they have either cut out of a magazine or down loaded from the web. How can we ever change this even if we want to?

What is not popularly circulated is the cost of acute innovations. The costs of new machinery have made a huge hole in budgets and in this way health is certainly a commodity. The reality, however, is that the social costs of pouring so much money into high-tech 'miracle' procedures have been enormous. Among the losers are large groups of the chronically ill, those living in rural and remote areas, socially and economically disadvantaged groups such as indigenous Australians, those with chronic mental illness, those with a developmental disability, and the frail elderly. As costs have risen in the acute end of the sector (where presently the majority of funds are spent) it is these groups who have been neglected, either through changes to the systems within which they were previously cared for, or through non-recognition of their increasing and different needs. As a direct result of modern technology and drug therapy we now have more chronically ill people in the community. Once they have left the acute sector they are abandoned to the system which exists outside the acute sector, where funds are scarce and the same level of discrete specialist knowledge may not be available. For these groups, health is a commodity they cannot afford.

5

THE PROBLEM OF EQUITY AND ACCESS

I was booked in as the first case for a minor procedure. The doctor came in and said in front of the waiting room, 'I can't do you because you're HIV positive and the operating theatre would be contaminated'. I was very vulnerable in an operating gown, sitting on a chair in public view. (R)

I have a friend who went to W hospital to have a bypass after three days in a peripheral hospital. After six days the doctor came in and said to him, 'How old are you?' and he said '73'. The doctor said to him: 'We'll give you some pills and send you home. You're 73; you can go home and potter in the garden.' (M)

If you've got an STD block on your phone, which most of us have, then you can't even ring the nearest medical practice [90 kilometres away] to book an appointment. If you can't do that then it is no good catching the bus because you can't get in to see him [the doctor]. Anyway the bus only goes into town once a week. Most days I haven't got the money to go into town—most of us live from fortnight to fortnight. (W)

The quotes above, taken from my recent discussions with patients, are just a few examples of the way in which people experience discrimination within the health care system. Indeed, the problem of equity and access constitutes one of the most significant issues for patients, and it is one which, while particular to a patient's situation, spans a variety of contexts and groups.

Access is defined in the 1999 NSW Department of Health Quality Framework document as: '. . . the extent to which an individual or population can obtain health care services. This often includes knowledge of when it is appropriate to seek health care, the ability to travel to and the means to pay for health care.'[1] This statement makes it clear that the present governmental notion of access does not mean that services will be available for all people but rather that services will be based on need. All communities across NSW cannot, for example, expect to have a cardiac catheter laboratory or even a hospital. But where there are clearly identified needs, such as a large aged population, then facilities (such as a nursing home) could be made available. Likewise, where there are increasing numbers of young families there may be a case for a baby health centre in a multipurpose centre which also organises immunisation, family and child health and counselling. Population size would determine whether it was viable to have such centres in a town or whether several communities could access facilities close by.

One of the fundamental problems in making a case about access to appropriate facilities and expertise lies in the narrow way in which access is defined by those who make decisions about health care funding. The issue of access usually focuses on hospitals and is often seen as reducible to waiting times. It is therefore measured on this basis, specifically in relation to services such as elective surgery, emergency, and outpatient services.[2] Clearly, however, for patients access is about much more than the amount of time spent waiting. Sometimes it is about not even getting the opportunity to wait, as will become clear later in this chapter, and as was the case with the elderly man at W hospital.

Not surprisingly, different individuals and groups experience different limitations in their ability to access adequate health care. While it is now well established that socioeconomic disadvantage is a major contributing factor to poorer health status,[3] it is also important to highlight the other factors that play a part. These factors may not be seen as disadvantages by those who tacitly block access for some patients by their attitudes, structures and practices.

So, while there are those for whom economic disadvantage is the main bar to adequate health care, others specifically identify

73

their social status as disadvantaging them, denying them access to health care similar in quality to those who may have a higher social status. Those trapped in poverty, either because of birth or unemployment, face a double jeopardy, suffering both social and economic disadvantage. Add to these factors the geographical isolation of those living in rural and remote communities, hours or even days from appropriate care, and there are individuals and entire communities who are severely disadvantaged relative to others in terms of their ability to access adequate health care.

Access to health care can also be limited by the physical parameters of a building, the availability of specialised expertise and/ or resources, and cultural forms of discrimination, which are expressed in the attitudes and practices of staff. Particularly affected are those who are mentally and physically disabled (for whom organised, publicly funded services have been dismantled over the past decades), the manual deaf (those who require sign language to comprehend), non-English speaking populations (whose access to information and decision-making is denied because of their inability to access culturally appropriate interpreters), and individuals whose health problems are regarded as a direct result of the way they live their lives (homosexual men who are HIV positive and drug-dependent men and women fall into this category).

It is also important to recognise that the acute illness focus of our present health care system also discriminates—specifically, against those with chronic illnesses in the community. For this group of patients, access to care is diminished because of the fact that the major percentage of health care funding is directed to acute illness which can be cured or which lends itself to surgical intervention—the high-tech end of health care. This highlights the aspect of discrimination which I believe to be the most concerning and most central to the future of our health as a nation. That is, vicarious discrimination through inequitable resource distribution.

This chapter attempts to articulate the complex problem of equity and access in the current system through an examination of a number of patients' stories and first-hand accounts of those who care for them. The stories have been gathered from individuals and groups as diverse as those living in rural communities where geographical isolation presents particular problems in relation to the accessing of health care; those living with the knowledge that they are HIV positive where issues are mostly about discrimination and access to up-to-date expertise; those with a disability such as deafness whose needs are poorly understood by professionals; those whose age prevents them from accessing adequate care; and indigenous Australians who are often at the greatest disadvantage due to a long and complex history of discriminatory practices.

DISCRIMINATORY PRACTICES

The 1960s were certainly not the halcyon days of equity and access or individualised care they are so often painted as being. Private patients were given very different care from the public patients, patients with mental illness or developmental disability were isolated from other patients, usually in separate institutions away from the city areas, and cancer was still a disease which elicited reactions which would now be perceived as ignorant. Unmarried mothers were hidden from the public gaze and their children removed for adoption because it was 'the best thing' for both mother and baby. I, and the vast majority of my colleagues, went along believing this was the case.

Perhaps my saddest memories are of the young girls who came into casualty after a backyard abortion. Many hospitals would not admit them and many staff avoided them. Without family or friends and labelled 'bad' by society, these girls died awful deaths because of overwhelming sepsis and severe haemorrhaging. Those who survived often lived with the guilt associated with their subsequent sterility. Now, when the abortion debate emerges once again, I think back to those individual girls and how it would have been so different for them today. They would have had choices, received more support, and experienced less discrimination.

There can be little argument about which group in Australia is the most generally disadvantaged due to past and present discriminatory practices, and who continue to be disadvantaged in gaining access to health care in all its aspects. Aboriginality is one of the major determinants of poor health status in Australia today, with up to twenty years' lower life expectancy in the Aboriginal than the non-Aboriginal population, as well as increased risk of heart disease, diabetes and fatal injury.[4] Contributing to the poor health status of indigenous Australians are the higher levels of unemployment, inadequate housing, lower levels of education and higher rates of incarceration they experience in both rural and city areas, factors which themselves can be understood as a result of discrimination.

When speaking about the status of her people's health at a recent national health conference, Puggy Hunter, a key Aboriginal spokesperson, lamented:

> . . . the basic human rights of the individual constantly are left behind when we talk about Aborigines. States have these human rights things . . . We have human rights to things like housing, rights to public health, Medicare, social security, social services and all these so-called international programs that Australia prides itself on signing off on. Makes you wonder [given the continuing state of Aboriginal health]. This [health] is about access: the right of us getting access to bring our people to the table.[5]

While much needs to be done, including the provision of significant resources targeted to correct huge anomalies in the living conditions of indigenous populations, at least by the end of the century there was some level of awareness among non-indigenous Australians of the structural inequities which have disadvantaged the indigenous population. In the 1960s there was limited, if any, awareness of the discrimination Aboriginal people were suffering. It certainly did not feature in our official documents or the rhetoric on health.

By the 1990s we at least had developed a separate National Aboriginal Health Strategy which clarifies the unique problems of this population. However, Stephen Leeder, who was part of the evaluation committee, has spoken of the culturally prejudiced attitudes that continue to stymie this strategy. As Leeder comments:

> While the view, that 'they' are ungrateful and dissolute, is maintained, the resulting political climate will mean that adequate resources will not be found to deal with these large issues that

need to be addressed through a comprehensive public health approach to Aboriginal health.[6]

Of course, when most people think about discrimination they think about attitudes and acts which are overtly directed towards a particular individual or group on the basis of obvious difference—because, for example, they're of a certain age, a certain sex, follow a particular religion, belong to a particular race or ethnic group, or have a disability. Direct discrimination, as this kind of discrimination is known by lawyers, is increasingly recognised as a problem in our community. The mechanics of direct discrimination are fairly straightforward. For example some people feel that there should be no priority accorded young people awaiting organ transplant.

But there's another, less recognised, form of discrimination which affects health care in Australia: indirect discrimination. Indirect discrimination happens when there's no intention to deny an individual a service, but they can't get access to it because of pre-existing inequities. If someone's told they're ineligible for a liver transplant because they're too old, then the discrimination would be direct. But if someone who lives in Dubbo was told they could only have a liver transplant if they have the resources to move to the inner city of Sydney and use the outpatient facilities there, then the discrimination would be indirect. Indirect discrimination is one of the major sources of inequity in our health care system today.

In the remainder of this chapter I want to look at two significant ways in which some Australians experience indirect discrimination —geographical isolation and communication limitations—and how they can severely limit their ability to access adequate health care services, particularly when compounded by direct discrimination, as it is for some.

ISOLATED COMMUNITIES

People living in isolated communities are particularly disadvantaged in relation to access to health care, although interestingly many will not necessarily identify themselves in this way. Disadvantage for this group is reflected in the recent demographic statistics on the health status of individuals and groups across Australia which show that the death rate for individuals in cities is lower than for those in large rural or remote areas. For example, men living in remote communities have a death rate four times greater than that of males living in capital cities. Their suicide rate reflects this trend, being 1.5 times the rate of men living in capital cities.[7]

There is also a higher incidence of cardiovascular disease in males in rural and remote areas, with the indigenous population being at greatest risk.[8] Indeed, between 1991 and 1995 death rates from all causes were greater for those living in rural and remote areas.[9] While lifestyle factors such as obesity, hypertension and smoking certainly contribute to such statistics, reduced access to health care, along with lower socioeconomic status, unemployment, less educational opportunity and a general feeling of low control over life, have also been shown to play a major role in this lower health status of people in rural communities.

In the past, most Australian rural communities were supported by a small hospital with a local general practitioner and bush nurse. Gradually these hospitals have been closed or turned into community or health centres and the town residents have been forced to travel to the nearest regional centres. In many such communities a nurse is available twenty-four hours a day with a general practitioner clinic held once or twice a week. One of the major problems presently being investigated is how to attract doctors to the country areas and how to keep them there. A downturn in the rural economy has seen many country towns reducing in size and losing their doctors. This has added to the inequities in access experienced by small rural communities.

Geographical location is a major factor, then, when it comes to accessing the same range and quality of services across the nation. A woman in an isolated rural community which relies mainly on ambulance services in emergencies, spoke about ringing the ambulance when she had severe vomiting, diarrhoea and abdominal pain. Because of the way in which she was treated she now feels frightened to go through the experience again, which in turn leaves her feeling even more isolated:

I had been sick all day and eventually rang the ambulance who took me into hospital at 2.00 a.m. Then I didn't see a doctor until 8.30 a.m. and he asked me why I had asked for an ambulance. It upset me so much I thought I must have done the wrong thing. He made me feel so guilty. If I didn't have an STD bar on my phone then I could have rung for telephone advice first, but now I'm frightened to call an ambulance.

If this woman had had access to some form of professional advice prior to calling the ambulance her experience might have been very different.

Access to adequate services is also difficult because of the state of the roads in some places. As C points out, 'We've got to drive 88 kilometres to the doctor over roads with potholes, so we've got to rely on nurses. We just sit and suffer because . . . we just can't get to the doctor.' This lack of geographical access makes it difficult for such people to manage even non-urgent medical problems. The nearest chemist to C is also nearly 100 kilometres away, making ready access to even the most simple medications impossible—even such medications as anti-fungal creams, pain-killers, and treatments for gastroenteritis (a common condition).

Compounding the problem of geographical isolation is the fact that many people in these communities are economically dis-advantaged, as patient W, a woman living in a rural community in NSW, explained at the beginning of this chapter.

Another woman in an isolated community whose daughter is on continuous antibiotic treatment for a urinary tract dysfunction also spoke with me about the structural problem she was experiencing in ensuring access to the drug:

Scripts run out and you have to wait until it finishes before you get a new script. Your health card only lasts one month and if you need to pay full price then you're nearly buggered unless you have a nurse around to negotiate with the doctor or the pharmacist.

Major emergencies also have their problems. R spoke about a neighbour who had her leg in plaster and rang her about it being cold: 'Her leg had signs of impaired circulation and the roads were cut off for cars. Anyway, I couldn't drive. The ambulance we rang needed directions to get from another town to ours which was over 200 kilometres.' As she spoke I remembered the recent furore during winter in the large city teaching hospitals as people were left waiting in city teaching hospital emergency departments for beds—'access block' it was called. There is no such thing in this community—there is simply no access.

The issue of access to expertise was raised by two women who, having searched for help in their immediate area, eventually came to a city specialist. One had a daughter with a reflux urethra. The daughter continued to have infection after infection. She had been to a general practitioner and a paediatrician in her local area without any change in her condition: 'Then I [the mother] went to the best [naming the doctor in Sydney]. I feel much better—I'm more at ease now she is on long-term antibiotics.' Another woman was married to a man with diabetes which he had suffered for thirty years but remained quite unstable: 'Finding someone within 200 kilometres with the expertise was the frustrating part.'

Others speak of how they managed without professional expertise in the past and thus have no expectations now. F and C, an elderly couple in an isolated rural setting, spoke of how they managed sickness over the years. Remembering a broken arm as a child C reflected, 'I had a broken arm . . . the headmaster set it and then I was taken to the doctor and he said, "Well I can't do any better than the headmaster's done." So it was left.'

In an effort to overcome access problems, communities become innovative and resourceful. One woman told me of her husband riding his pushbike home after he had a snake bite and how a group orchestrated his care. She went on: 'The next-door neighbour put the bandage on—she knows how to do it, and then J drove us to hospital because she can drive.' This raised the issue of a community taking control of their own health, by making sure the necessary skills and knowledge were available among members of the community, thus compensating for their lack of access.

Individuals in such areas have undertaken First Aid certificates and one group had even raised money for an Oxy Viva unit, which delivers oxygen used in resuscitation. Of course, the solution is not as simple as just having high-tech equipment. As M said:

> You need to have someone willing to take responsibility for the Oxy Viva unit because something has to be done while you're waiting for the ambulance (which might be hours away). And the unit needs to be checked and maintained. Emergencies are touch and go here.

In keeping with the Australian experience generally, the isolated communities which are most disadvantaged are Aboriginal ones. J, a community nurse who had spent many years working and living in an isolated Aboriginal community, spoke with me about her experiences, about the close links she felt with the people there, along with the frustrations and challenges she faced as a nurse. J was accepted as part of the community, she lived there, had her children there and found it difficult to leave when the time came.

COMMUNICATION

Communication issues are another common source of indirect discrimination, both for people who speak a primary language other than English and for those with low literacy skills. Literacy includes not only the ability to read but in some cases to comprehend both written and verbal messages, particularly those which use technical jargon or sophisticated language. A lack of literacy can leave many feeling helpless—unable to comprehend information or to negotiate the administrative aspects of the health care system. Of course, low literacy levels are directly related to lower socioeconomic levels, a factor which further compounds these patients' problems. As S, who can't write, explains: 'I find it very difficult to write a letter when I have to explain about my Medicare card. I have to pay up-front for the specialist in the nearest town and it costs $100 before you can claim it back.' The nurse in this community usually writes the letters for patients if they need to explain why they are unable to pay for a specialist visit. She also initiated literacy and computer classes for the community so that they could feel more in control.

Another major group who attract discrimination are non-English speakers. It's not just a matter of being able to understand signs—there's the problem that services have been set up in a way which is often fundamentally different to how things are done in their country of origin. Lack of cultural awareness among service planners and providers means that health services are not used as fully as they could be. This has become an increasingly pressing issue in Australia where there are now a large number of ethnic groups often requiring special services. In 1996, 2.5 million Australians, aged 5 years old and over, spoke a language other than English at home. Of these, 74 per cent were born overseas and 22 per cent were the children of those born overseas.[10] It has been shown that, in general, immigrants have better health than the Australian-born population when they arrive (their original health status may have something to do with entry criteria) but that it deteriorates over time.[11]

Of course, like all groups, the non-English speaking population is not homogenous and so their health status differs according to their country of origin. To enable access to services, interpreters have been made available by federal funding and some state funding, but these are not always well coordinated nor accessible to all requiring them. There is also anecdotal evidence that cost constraints have meant a cutting of such services.[12] Therefore, along with feeling alienated due to cultural differences, individuals who are unable to communicate in English are also severely disadvantaged in our English-speaking health care system with a workforce trained and immersed in a 'Westernised bio-medical culture'.[13]

Another group with reduced access due to communication differences are the deaf, particularly those who depend on lip reading along with either speech or sign language. While those born with a sensorineural deafness today benefit from technological advances such as hearing aids and cochlear implants, as well as from the giant steps made in educational techniques, there are several generations of deaf people who were brought up without the benefit of such advances. For many of those people the only option is to communicate through a combination of sign language and lip reading.

The lack of awareness in general about the effect of deafness on learning has left its legacy in terms of inadequate literacy levels for many who are now adults. This disadvantages them in numerous ways, including inability to communicate outside their group without the assistance of a sign language interpreter, inability to access anything more than the most basic literature on health matters, inability to communicate in an informed way with health professionals, feelings of low esteem, alienation and frustration, and even unemployment. These disadvantages are all evident in the following stories.

D, a profoundly deaf young man from birth who is in his thirties, has undertaken tertiary studies and has a senior position with a major banking institution. He spoke with me recently about his experiences with the health care system. He had quite a bit to say about general practitioners:

> It's only in the last years I have had a GP who treated me like an individual. He didn't sort of try to patronise me in any way. He certainly made no assumptions about whether I understood the information he gave me. He would explain it to me. He took his time. The GPs I have had before . . . who I sensed were talking to me in a very degrading way . . . talked to me as if I had the intellectual ability of a 12 year old . . . they wouldn't explain what medicine I was taking or how it was working or why I should take it. In one case a GP spoke to me in such a way . . . that it was very simplistic childish language. I came out feeling 'I'll never go back to him again'. I had gone to him because the last GP I went to was so bad. Something I have never been able to understand is if I am communicating with someone in an adult way why they can't communicate with me in a normal way. It is something my current GP does do. I would say that he has had something to do with aged deafness because he looked after a whole village of elderly people and that is why he is so good.

More recently he had a very positive health experience; however, it was limited to a very specialised unit within a private hospital. All the patients were coming in for cochlea implantation and all were deaf. As a result the unit and staff were specially chosen and trained to deal with this group of patients. As he said, 'I had none of the usual problems faced by deaf people'.

I also spoke with a young deaf woman, J, who was born deaf and relies on signing and lip reading. She has had three children and lost a child at thirteen months. She began with her recent experience in childbirth only five months previously:

> It was really good because I had an interpreter coming regularly to visit me. X hospital have a lot of deaf women coming to their hospital so they have a great service . . . When R [her third baby] was born I didn't have an interpreter with me and my husband interpreted for me. The midwives would say 'push', my husband would tell me to push. But it was when the midwife was giving me stitches I wanted to complain because it was hurting. I was screaming but I was signing and I had a gas mask on. But the midwife said 'Oh I've only got two more to go' and it seemed like she wanted to ignore me and just get on with it. And my husband said to her to stop. 'She needs more anaesthetic.' But the midwife seemed that she just wanted to finish. So she hurried and finished. Then the midwife said 'Sorry' but I was crying and upset and couldn't stop crying. Later my mother came and asked what was wrong and I told her. And my mother wrote a letter but I said forget it . . . it's just not worth sending it. I just don't want to go through the bad memories. I just want to forget it.

J went on to describe her experience of losing her child and her inability to access information about the death:

> When my daughter died it was really important to have an interpreter but I couldn't get an interpreter because none were available. You really need an interpreter when this happens. The doctor gave me lots of notes but I couldn't understand his notes, the terminology he used. He said my daughter had a fit. At the moment I don't know why she died. When she died she had to have an autopsy. They said she died from pneumonia but I said 'No, she died from a cot death'. But they said she was too old for a cot death. But she wasn't sick, she was happy and playing before she went to bed.

All in all, within this group of people who were deaf from birth, some who were oral and some who relied on a signed interpreter, there was considerable consensus on their major needs. And these needs were basic. They wanted to be able to communicate and to be able to do that in their own language whether that was through sign language and lip reading, speaking and lip reading or appropriate technology such as a teletypewriter (TTY). The central element in all the stories, however, was the need to be treated with respect as an individual who counted. And this may mean that the doctor or nurse needed to take a little more time to ensure an interpreter was available and that they spoke in a way which enabled lip reading by the patient. In some of the stories I was told there was also clear evidence that informed consent was not obtained for several procedures, raising questions around duty of care issues. Surely this is an added imperative for professionals to ensure that truly informed consent has been obtained using whatever means is required.

DISTRIBUTION OF SERVICES

At the heart of any adequate health care system is the ability of the people to access some form of health care. One of the disadvantages most people expect when choosing to live in small rural and remote communities is the lack of access to the same level of health care as those living in cities. What they do need and expect, however, is 24-hour access to basic professional expertise—doctor, nurse, or preferably both—supplied by people who understand the context in which they live. They also expect professionals to be supportive and competent. The facilities they want are those which best suit the needs of the particular community. In an ageing community this might be an aged care facility with respite care and in most communities the requirement is for a community health centre and a rapid response to emergencies in terms of triage and transport. There is now a move towards multipurpose centres in small communities which take the place of a hospital, but with fewer beds as well as providing primary health care across the life span.

The key factors in all this are equity in terms of access, and a sense of fair play in terms of budget allocation. While the major proportion might go to the large teaching hospitals, this would be acceptable if communities perceive that they are being treated fairly in terms of their share of public funding. In some cases, this might mean better funding of non-health services. As Stephen Leeder points out:

> ... the investment of capital and other national wealth for productive non-health purposes may do more for health than spending it on hospitals and doctors' fees ... Creating employment opportunities for members of Aboriginal communities may also be health enhancing as well as giving them a secure economic base.[14]

This was confirmed by the Health Education Officer at an Aboriginal Community Centre in rural NSW. The Centre is run by a corporation consisting of Aboriginal people who also live on the land. They have purchased a property through a community development program and intend to grow wheat and be self-sustaining. As A told me:

> We provide employment for local people from the community and a couple from surrounding towns. Give them work. Give them something to do. Mainly 15 hours a week and they get paid in return. Initially it was the equivalent of working for the dole but what we try to do is give them a 38 hour week and put them on a traineeship. What it comes down to is self-esteem. If you're working you feel better about yourself.

The community supports its own health program including women's health, nutrition and sexually transmitted disease education programs. The young people are encouraged to take up sport and while there are drug problems these are controlled by the community itself. They have also linked with their nearest university in a project to grow bush tucker. A spoke of how such strategies are turning individuals and families around:

> There were a lot of people who were on insulin and are off it now ... changing the diet. We're up-to-date with everything here. Immunisations, and screenings. B has a vehicle to take

people to their appointments. When I started work the ladies here were very frightened. Now when their appointments come up they are there.

Presently, distribution of the national health care dollar is inequitable if one considers what the major health problems are in our communities. While the bulk of funding is consumed by hospitals with 38 per cent, medical services with 20 per cent and pharmaceuticals with 12 per cent, community and public health services are way behind with only 4 per cent of the funding.[15] Yet the major health problems are not those which lead to hospitalisation. These include hypertension, respiratory infections, diabetes, back complaints, osteoarthritis and psychiatric disorders such as depression. The majority of these are chronic problems while drug dependency is also becoming a major health problem. General practitioners manage the bulk of the health problems of our society, maintaining people outside hospitals, while the major proportion of resources is spent on hospital care. Of course, the federal funding of general practitioners and the state funding of hospitals make it difficult to compare resource distribution accurately. But increasingly the cost of maintaining hospitals is causing governments to look for alternative methods of funding, such as moving more resources to the private sector to relieve the pressure on the public sector.

Given the direct links between poverty and health status through factors such as housing, clean water, sanitation, nutrition, education, self-esteem and a sense of well-being, we need to look at the issue of equity more generally if we are to address the specific problem of health care equity. Fran Baum, a speaker at the 5th National Rural Health Conference, highlighted the UNICEF/WHO report showing that 'the world's 358 billionaires have a combined net worth of $US760 billion which is equal to the total assets of the poorest 45% of the world's population'.[16] Paralleling this global trend, in Australia there is evidence that there is an increasing gap between those who are identified as super rich (incomes of $500 000+ a year) and those who are on low incomes (less than $25 000 a year). A healthy Australia surely depends on well-supported communities—supported by structures, resources and policies ensuring equitable access to a healthy life in all its permutations.

We need to be more vigilant about the various ways in which discrimination manifests itself. In relation to health care, many past practices have now been exposed as discriminatory. Today, Australians are, on balance, more likely to be made to reflect on their own values and assumptions both because of increased access to information and because of legislation designed to protect against discrimination, but this in and of itself does not overcome entrenched values and beliefs. So, despite an increased awareness of the nature of our cultural prejudices and the enactment of legislation to protect those disadvantaged by such attitudes, discrimination continues. We can only hope to monitor practices carefully and to put in place structures which support groups who have been discriminated against because of a lack of services, insensitive attitudes and cultural practices, incompetence, indifference and lack of education or finance. Ultimately, discrimination needs to be exposed and eradicated through a more transparent system which critiques individual practices along with system-wide practices. But, even with the most open system possible, equity ultimately depends on services being available, funded and distributed in a way which takes into account the specific needs of all individuals and groups.

6

DESIGNING HEALTH CARE

At least it gives our people a sense of dignity about going to the doctor, because if you abolish it we have to go cap in hand and some of us are too bloody proud for that. And we've got to fight the rich and powerful sources ready to sink Medicare and the public health system.

As B spoke passionately about his concerns I looked around the group I had spent the morning with. They were all members of the Pensioners and Superannuants Group, having lived and worked through the years of changes I have discussed in this book. They epitomised informed consumers and told me how vulnerable they now felt whenever it seemed that Medicare was to be removed. They were fierce about hanging on to their independence in whatever way they could, having made a huge contribution to society during their paid working days and now continuing that in a voluntary capacity as advocates for all pensioners and superannuants. Their sense of personal and community responsibility is stronger than ever, making a mockery of the current political rhetoric that social benefits breed dependence. Indeed, they were one of the most informed and proactive groups I met.

There is no doubt that the organisation, management and funding of health care is one of the contemporary dilemmas for Western nations. Given the advances in medical science, specifically the sophisticated surgical techniques which make what were once major and even risky procedures more accessible and attractive, as well as the increase in and ageing of our population, it is understandable that the demands on our health care system are increasing daily. As a result, governments world-wide are developing alternative designs and models of care which can continue to provide the best of health care to as many as possible within increasingly constrained budgets.

In Australia, models of care delivery have come and gone according to the changing social, cultural and political climate. Some are driven by governments for economic purposes (such as user pays models), some by consumers (such as the women's health model), while many are developed and driven by practitioners to meet the special needs of patients or communities (such as the various community practitioner models). While technology itself drives much of what nurses now do in critical care areas, primary care models in isolated areas have been developed to facilitate greater equity and access in communities where more needs to be done with less.

This chapter describes the broad framework of health care currently in place in Australia, as well as alternative models of care. In particular, I examine the cultural and political ideology driving the system and reflected through funding models, resource distribution, organisational management across sectors, and the way in which care is delivered to individuals and populations. Present models of care delivery are explored along with the historical and ideological context which gave rise to them. This examination of the current macro and micro levels of system organisation then provides the context within which potential future models of care can be envisioned and evaluated.

CURRENT SYSTEMS

Health care systems across the world are set up and managed in a variety of ways. For example, the USA has a predominantly private system, the UK a universally-funded public system, while Canada has what some describe as a publicly funded private system.[1] Canada's is perhaps closest to Australia's health care system in that it is funded through personal taxation, but differs in that it does not have the layers of government involvement, and medical fees are capped.

In Australia, we have a mixed public/private health care system, although ours is still predominantly a public system with 11 per cent of our total health expenditure supporting private health insurance.[2] The system is complicated in the way it is structured and funded because of the division between federal and state governments and bureaucracies. While the major financial commitment by the federal government is the funding of the public hospitals through the Commonwealth Medicare Agreement with the states ($30.2 billion over five years in 1998), it also provides a subsidy for private health insurance ($1.7 billion over three years in 1998), pharmaceutical benefits payments and special projects such as vaccination or anti-smoking programs and Aboriginal and Torres Strait Islander health initiatives.[3] General practitioner rebates and projects are also funded by the federal government, as are residential aged care facilities.

So not only is there a public/private mix in the distribution of funding, access and management of care, the system is further complicated by the federal/state government divide which affects the structures and policies. To add to this complex configuration, local governments also have a role to play, mainly in the area of community services and disease prevention and public health.

The Department of Health and Family Services is the federal government body which administers Medicare, our universal scheme of health care insurance, funded nationally through indexed personal taxation. The federal government not only allocates funds to the states for public hospitals through a five-year negotiated Medicare agreement, it also pays for community-based medical services and subsidises pharmaceutical and residential aged care facilities. Medicare also reimburses patients for a proportion of the cost of services provided by qualified medical practitioners, eligible dental practitioners and optometrists, through a scheme in which there is a predetermined schedule of fees. Medical care in a public hospital, as well as the accommodation, is also covered under Medicare.

Despite the schedule of fees set under Medicare, medical practitioners are not required to comply with this set schedule; their fees are not capped, which in some cases results in gaps which patients are required to meet over and above their contribution through taxation.[4] Approximately 30 per cent of the Australian community take out private insurance to address this gap and to be able to access private hospital care and other services such as dental care, therapies and appliances not covered by Medicare. But even this does not necessarily eliminate the gap payment. Numbers taking out private insurance declined considerably as the gap between medical fees and private insurance rebates increased throughout the 1990s, leaving the privately insured patient with bills over and above those reimbursed by their insurance. Presently, the federal government and insurance companies are attempting to address this through incentive schemes to attract people back to the private schemes and thus relieve the pressure on the public system.[5]

State governments' main fiscal responsibility is the public hospital system through the funding they receive from the Commonwealth Medicare Agreement (which is now known as the Australian Health Care Agreement), which currently runs from July 1998 until June 2003. Increasingly this agreement has been contentious and in 1998 the majority of states initially refused to sign off on the agreement for the next five years because of the insufficiency of funding to meet the changing needs of the system. While the federal government claimed they had increased funding by 15 per cent over the five years, the states were not convinced of the fairness of the agreement, given that they had the responsibility for service delivery and effectiveness of outcomes. As Dr John Hewson writes in the *Australian Financial Review*:

> Putting ego and petulance aside, health funding is a crucial issue and goes to the very heart of the Commonwealth–State fiscal imbalance. The Commonwealth provides the cash, the States do the spending and provide the service. The Commonwealth claims a 15 percent increase but the States have to adjust for demographic factors, the aging of the population and the requirements of service delivery—the 15 percent becomes 1 percent, insufficient to deliver what patients now demand.[6]

Another federal government service is the Home and Community Care (HACC) program providing for frail aged and younger disabled people not in residential care. There has, however, been a gradual shift to the consumer being charged a certain amount for many of these services according to ability to pay. In addition to this shift towards user pays, the amount spent on nursing homes has decreased—despite the ageing of the population—thus making it difficult for many people to access nursing home care if they do not have the means to buy into a private nursing home. Meanwhile, funding to the acute sector has increased[7] while at the same time funding to aged care has diminished in real terms.

Our present system of funding pharmaceuticals is also at some risk of erosion as it becomes an increasing burden on our health care budget.[8] Presently the federal Health Insurance Commission administers the Pharmaceutical Benefits Scheme providing subsidised, and therefore affordable, drugs to many Australians. The Pharmaceutical Benefits Advisory Committee (PBAC) evaluates each new drug in relation to its clinical and cost effectiveness through comparisons with similar drugs on the market, and as a result of their gate-keeping role they are under constant attack from drug companies. The massive increase in drugs coming on to the market makes this scheme vital in terms of managing what is an increasingly unmanageable drug company bonanza with its inevitable costs to the community.

While there are differences in the structuring of health care across the states and territories in Australia, it is these governments which have the major responsibility for the provision of public health care. They do this primarily through public hospitals, including psychiatric hospitals, and community public health programs. More recently, acute psychiatric services have been incorporated into specific public hospitals, with smaller group accommodation or community-based centres also available for those with mental health problems. There are also community-based crisis teams to meet the growing needs of those now living in the community with some form of mental illness. Child, adolescent and family health services, women's health, some dental health services, home and community care, and rehabilitation services are also the responsibility of state and territory governments, along with the regulation of health service premises and personnel.

Given that the states and territories need to manage the increasing demand for health care in hospitals yet have only minimal control over the proportion of funding they receive from the federal government, there is a level of frustration and tension over this separation of funding and management. Five-yearly 'negotiated funding' battles become increasingly confrontational as the pressure on the health care system increases from all stakeholders, with each government refusing to accept responsibility for the funding cuts.

It is clear that managing the health care of our nation is a complicated matter because of the various sectorial interests involved, the structures which need to be established and funded, the policies which need to be developed and monitored, and the personnel who require education and training. And, finally, there is the matter of evaluating practices to ensure that what is in operation actually meets the health needs of the population, is accessible to those who need it, and leads to a healthy nation. When all this occurs in a setting like Australia, where federal and seven state/territory governments each have their own agendas for managing and funding the system, it is no wonder that individuals are confused about how to access the system and that governments are confused about which pressures to heed and which to ignore. After all, these pressures usually come from groups or individuals wanting additional funding.

In addition to understanding the 'how' of funding when analysing any system of health care, it is important to also take into account the 'why' behind decisions about resource distribution. Specifically, it is important to consider the general ideological model of health assumed by governments and others with decision-making powers. For example, when it comes to the funding of our present health system, it seems that a narrow, biomedical, illness-focused model has been employed, with the emphasis on illness and cure rather than on health and prevention. This is reflected in the structures that are implemented, the way resources are distributed, how research is funded and contexts of care that are valued.

RESOURCE DISTRIBUTION

The way in which resources are distributed provides particular evidence of an illness focus, with tertiary care funded far above primary health care. In 1995–96 we spent 38.1 per cent of our recurrent health expenditure on hospitals, 20.2 per cent on medical services, 7.6 per cent on nursing homes, and an unavailable figure on community and public health, although this was 5.2 per cent in

1993-94.[9] Given that the most frequently reported ailments include respiratory problems such as asthma and bronchitis, cardiovascular ones such as hypertension and heart disease, and musculoskeletal disorders such as back problems and arthritis,[10] and taking into account the more basic health problems which continue to affect our most disadvantaged groups, the emphasis on funding acute services surely requires review. While some of these conditions may result in hospital admission, in the main they are not curable but are managed most appropriately through public health strategies such as nutritional and exercise programs, early prevention and diagnosis, education on self-management, and support through better community services.

Our present health care system appears also to have ignored the established link between socioeconomic status and health outcome measures.[11] The first research report of the National Health Strategy in 1992, investigating inequalities in the basic health of different groups in our community, showed that:

. . . Overall standardised death rates are highest for those from areas experiencing the worst socioeconomic disadvantage. Compared with people from advantaged areas, these people have standardised death rates which range from being 46 per cent higher (for girls) to 67 per cent higher (for men).[12]

It has also been shown that those with limited economic resources also access preventive services less than those who have greater resources, despite the fact that they may need them more than others. If we took such factors into account in terms of evidence on which to evaluate our services, then we might be funding programs which link our present health care system with other sectors including housing, sanitation, nutrition, education and employment, to ensure a more primary health, preventive focus.

On the United Nations Human Development Index, which measures a nation's level of social and economic inequality, Australia has now slipped from seventh to fifteenth place,[13] a fact which should be setting off alarm bells for all of us since poverty is a key indicator of poor health status. We know there are now an increasing number of Australians at risk of poorer health because they live in poverty (11.5 per cent of our population compared with 8.2 per cent in 1973) yet little, if anything, is done for such groups when health priorities are set. Somehow this falls outside the health portfolio, perhaps because of the complexity it presents.

One of the more contentious aspects of our present system of funding is the waste and cost shifting promoted by the public–private and Commonwealth–state splits. Examples of cost shifting are increasing as the deliverers of health care respond to financial, social and political changes. For example, as reduced funding to residential aged care has led to cuts in staffing numbers and skill mix, residents of nursing homes (federally funded) are referred to emergency departments of public hospitals (state funded) for minor procedures such as catheter reinsertion, once handled in nursing homes. This situation has been compounded by many general practitioners being unwilling to attend nursing homes citing workload, changed hours of work and what they regard as inadequate financial reimbursement. This is compounded by policies that assuage the interest of particular constituencies to the disadvantage of others—surely the antithesis of effective management. While such divides exist, our health care system will remain inefficient and, more importantly, not focused on the needs of either individuals or society. It will therefore never right the present and increasing inequities as far as funding and therefore access are concerned.

CURRENT MODELS OF CARE

Given our relatively inequitable and complex health care system, a diverse range of models of care delivery have been developed to overcome some of the problems facing patients in accessing effective care. Indeed, despite, or perhaps to compensate for, the fact that our present national framework of health care is focused on illness, some practitioners focus on preventing illness, promoting healthy lifestyles and encouraging individuals to take responsibility for their own health. These models are of particular importance in isolated communities where individuals need to be more self-sufficient in terms of managing their own health and illness because of the lack of easy access to health care professionals or facilities. Despite such diversity, in the main health care in Australia is still delivered within traditional models largely driven by the institution and/or health professional rather than the patient.

When I began nursing there was only one model of care as far as I can remember, and it was definitely practitioner driven. The 1960s was an era in which illness was still viewed as deviant and alienating, and medicine and nursing were seen as beneficent practices. This perspective placed both professions in the role of moral guardians of society, their function being to control deviance (illness). Hospitals were structured in a way that suited the doctors and nurses rather than the patients, placing patients in a disempowered position. They were expected to be compliant and submissive, and were often left feeling guilty if they did not get better (see Chapter 1). Patients were the last to know anything, even their diagnosis or prognosis. In such an environment we practised what was known as task centred care.

Task centred care involved tasks being allocated according to the level of the nurse, measured in terms of years of experience. In first year we did the cleaning of bodies and furniture, as well as attending to all the bodily needs of the patients who were mainly bed bound. Halfway through first year we might be trusted to take temperatures, count respirations, and even measure blood pressures. Second year saw us move up the pecking order to give out drugs, and finally in third year we could at last dress wounds. Such allocation of tasks mitigated against our developing any rapport with a patient as we moved rapidly from bed to bed measuring, counting, and recording. In third year if a wound was particularly complex, then we might have the opportunity for a conversation with the patient. Doctors' rounds were also done with military precision; the specialist and charge sister led an entourage of students from bed to bed as charts were consulted, wounds were inspected and students were interrogated. Only rarely was the patient involved beyond a token 'How are you today?'. In the main, patients did not speak to the doctor during rounds. Interestingly, task centred care may be alive and well in our system today, perhaps due to the cost-cutting which has meant fewer registered nurses in the system with a greater turnover of patients.

While patients in the 1960s remained passive in terms of being part of the decision-making about their care, changes were evident in the 1970s as a few patients began to question decisions. We were moving into the age of knowledge sharing which was gradually to shift power towards the patients. Of course, in the community the models of care were always more patient-centred since community nurses were reliant on patients allowing them access to their environments as they made home visits. I can well remember having lectures on the difference between caring for a patient in a hospital and in their own home. Nevertheless, the difference was not great as far as the relationship was concerned, with the patient still deferring to the nurse and doctor. This began to change around the 1970s, with the women's movement playing a major part in one of the first patient-driven models of care.

Women's health models were driven by women themselves, who demanded the right to be cared for by women. In NSW one of the first Women's Health Centres was established in Leichhardt in 1974. H, who worked there as a women's health nurse, remembers, 'This model of care originally arose out of an activist ideology—a move to make things happen and not just live in the rhetoric.'

Women's health centres slowly began to be established in other states. W spoke to me about the excitement of being able to set up this model of care in the ACT because of the support of the Minister of Health, Dr Neal Blewett. She had 'incredible support' in her new role working with a variety of health care workers including an Aboriginal health worker, an interpreter for women whose first language was not English, and later a staff member who learned sign language so she could speak with women who were deaf.

The women's health model is also an example of a multi-disciplinary or interdisciplinary model of care. Multidisciplinary care is a patient-centred model of care since it focuses on a specific population or group of patients, and is not necessarily centred on the health professionals like other models of care. This has been the traditional model in community mental health teams and more recently in the care of the elderly, with Aged Care Assessment Teams available for assessment of the needs of the elderly, either in their home or in a hospital setting. Within this model the focus is on the skills of each person in the team regardless of their discipline or profession and how these skills can best strengthen the team. Palliative care, particularly in the community, is also carried out by multidisciplinary teams, although in the main nurses carry out the actual hands-on care and counselling in the home. And increasingly, general practitioners are delivering services using a diverse group of practitioners ranging from nurses, chiropractors, acupuncturists, physiotherapists and psychologists.

Multidisciplinary or interdisciplinary care has, therefore, the capacity to facilitate the sharing of different disciplinary perspectives, encouraging care which focuses the team on the needs of the patient and family rather than on those of the practitioners. In hospitals, despite such advantages and despite the fact that patients are cared for by a range of professionals, there is limited attention to truly multidisciplinary models of care.

Focusing on the patient and family is also an aspect of primary care. Perhaps the best example of this was the traditional family doctor, and there are signs of a return to this model—it was so effective. General practice groups have moved to calling their practices 'family medicine'. The family doctor of the past was a respected friend and confidant of the family from birth until death. He (the doctor was typically male although this is not presently the case) not only delivered the babies, he looked after these babies throughout their lives, even to the point of delivering their babies. He was on call 24 hours a day and was able to move from the home to the hospital if necessary. He was the one who organised a hospital bed if it was needed, and he might even do the surgery. This model was driven more by the context of the time than by the patient, but today it would be welcomed back by those who remember it. Many older people I interviewed shared fond memories of their family doctor. The model might even address the problem of the fragmentation of care we now face, despite the advantages of specialisation.

In the 1970s a plethora of models emerged to overcome the mechanistic approach of the task centred nursing care of the 1960s. One such model was primary nursing, driven not only by patients receiving long-term palliative care who preferred to have a nurse they could contact 24 hours a day, but also by nurses who found task centred care very unrewarding. Senior hospital management supported this model since the emerging focus on quality assurance demanded greater attention to patients' needs and satisfaction. In primary nursing patients were allocated a registered nurse when they were admitted and that nurse looked after them during their time in hospital and at times even after discharge.

Evaluations of this model showed high levels of satisfaction for both patient and nurse. Eventually, as the economists gained greater power in the system, this model was viewed as too expensive and a derivation appeared called team nursing, in which a group of patients are nursed by a team of nurses of varying levels of expertise. This is the way in which many hospital wards are managed at present since it adjusts for the fact that not all nurses are registered nurses but are all expected to provide direct care. Team nursing enables a registered nurse to manage the allocation and supervision of care among the team as well as being directly involved in the care.

Primary or one-to-one nursing was also a necessary model in the newly established intensive care units of the 1970s and 1980s since the majority of patients were ventilated. While primarily patient-centred, this model of care was driven by issues of safety since nurses were working with sophisticated technology in restructured specialist wards where the focus was on the miracles performed by the specialists. While this did mean that more lives were saved, the move to specialist practice also meant the gradual demise of the family doctor. Specialisation added another layer in the system, a costly layer and one which grows daily as new diseases are named which require new specialists to manage them, new drugs to be discovered, and new units to be built. The specialist model of care is the major one used in today's acute health care sector.

A new model of care, which aims to address gaps in health care in rural and remote areas, is that of the Nurse Practitioner, which was legislated for in NSW in 1998. This model is community driven as well as a natural evolution in health care as nurses have become more highly educated and skilled in diagnosing and managing increasingly complex health care problems. A Nurse Practitioner will be an advanced level nurse working in an extended role in a specific context, thereby addressing the special needs of a group of patients. This has the potential to overcome fragmentation of care and indeed, like several other models, it has characteristics similar to the family doctor model of care where there was a central figure who managed care for the whole family. Many nurses working in isolated communities with only limited access to medical support are already providing such care, as well as integrating care across all sectors of the community by attending to the housing, employment and education needs of families. And in most cases they are on call 24 hours a day.

Juxtaposed against such patient- and community-focused models are other contemporary models which reflect the recent trend of treating health as a commodity. Early discharge and day only surgery are models of care which have arisen out of the move to commodify health, although both may have their advantages in that they avoid what has become an unsafe environment—the hospital. Early discharge, while more a mechanism for managing the demands on the system, also dictates the way in which care needs to be carried out, so in this way it is a model of care. Over the last decade there has been a strategic plan to reduce the length of stay in hospital for patients undergoing surgery or following childbirth and, to this end, early discharge protocols and procedures have been implemented. This has required new ways of assessing patients prior to surgery, such as pre-admission clinics which reduce the need for patients to be admitted the night before surgery and help to plan for discharge with the patient prior to admission. In this way the patient and relatives can plan for their shortened length of stay in hospital and their care after discharge.

Hospital in the home is a model that works to reduce hospital stay by caring for patients in their homes. This involves selecting appropriate patients—that is, those who do not necessarily require specialist care or constant vigilance and who feel comfortable staying in their own homes during their episode of illness. Care is managed through the Area Health Services with practitioners supplied by the hospital or the local general practitioner practice. In some instances hospital in the home may require costly technology, such as a ventilator, but given that patients have been undergoing renal dialysis at home for many years, this is not really new, although the naming of the model is.

THE IMPACT OF CURRENT MODELS ON PATIENTS

How have the various models of care described above affected patients' lives? And how well do they meet the needs of a population? Initially I inquired about models that have been mainly driven by practitioners—in other words, those practices which are designed primarily to meet the needs of the professional. D talked to me of her recent experience in a hospital as she underwent spinal surgery:

> Because I was a public patient I went to the admission clinic. They were all registered nurses and it was very task oriented. I thought it would be mind numbing to work down there because you were taking blood pressures from every patient. But from a patient's point of view it was quite good because you got all this stuff done without having to go into hospital the night before.

But, as D revealed, what appeared to be an efficient and cost-effective model of care for surgical patients was somehow negated when all the measurements and tests were repeated on admission the next day: 'There's obviously a lack of faith there somewhere or continuity of care or something.'

The specialist model of care, which now dominates the acute health care system, has led to care which patients experience as fragmented. Patients speak about how they are merely seen as a hand, a shoulder or a liver, and how they have no one who sees them as a person. As A said to me as we sat in the Hand Clinic at a major referral hospital, 'When the doctor comes out I am sure he looks around and sees hands rather than people on the seats'. D also spoke about her experience in a neurosurgical unit after major spinal surgery:

> So my major interaction with the nursing staff was that I asked for pain relief and they gave it to me. Apart from that I really had no interactions with the nursing staff. They would come in, they would redo the drip, they would give me antibiotics—so it was really a drug-related interaction with the nursing staff.

Perhaps the most contentious issue arising from the move to specialist models of care, however, is that of funding. For C it was central to her management in a private hospital:

> First of all his [the orthopaedic surgeon's] receptionist called me the day before and she told me that if I didn't come in to pre-pay the surgeon's fee I would not be admitted to the hospital. So the night before I was to have surgery on my knee I walked to his clinic three blocks from a parking place. So it was a very inflamed knee when I went into hospital. For hospital fees and the room staying overnight it was $1400 and the surgeon was $1000 or something. So I'd already paid that before I'd got to my room.

M spoke to me about the ill-will created by all the bills he received after surgery, bills he had not expected:

> When I had my hernia operated on the second assistant to the surgeon sent me a bill for $48.00. I didn't pay him because I didn't know who he was. If he had said hello before I went in and said, 'I'm Bill Smith's assistant and I'll be holding your tube up' then I would have paid the bill in a snap.

M went on:

> Unless people make a contract with me by shaking my hand or looking me in the eye and explaining what they are going to do and what they are going to charge me for, I really don't want to pay. It happened again when we got a bill from the paediatrician that was quite unannounced [recently he and his wife also had a baby]. It wasn't explained by our obstetrician as that's what was going to happen, and he was there for about 30 seconds and A [their daughter] is a public patient in a public hospital—so why were they milking us for all they could? Because we bought a $2000 chunk of time from a private obstetrician it then contaminated us.

His wife S commented:

> And there are heaps of bills we got for pathology for all sorts of bits and pieces that we were never told we would have to pay

for. I just thought I would have to pay for my visits to the obstetrician. Over $1000 of bills for tests that had been done, and if I had been a public patient I would never have had to pay . . .

This process of a specialist using the services of one or more extra specific specialists during the episode of care for which he has been contracted is a common one. These specialists, who may not have even met the patient, will forward their bills to the patient after the procedure. While not specifically a model of care it is nevertheless part of the way in which specialist care is managed and funded within the private system.

The lack of access to specialist health care in country areas is currently a criticism by rural communities and the doctors who work there. For the doctors this means demanding high Medicare rebates which in turn creates difficulties for patients who are required to pay up-front fees, which many are unable to do. The rural doctors justify such charges as due to the 'higher costs they face and the demand made of them for broader skills. They work longer hours, travel more and have to use a wide range of skills including anaesthetics, surgery and psychiatry because of the absence of specialists nearby.'[14]

But there are those for whom the lack of specialist units is not perceived as a disadvantage. K, who spent five years flying back and forth to a major city hospital with her daughter, saw the advantage of locating super specialist units in major city hospitals where practice is based on the very latest research and specialist doctors, and where nurses learn and practice together, rather than in isolation. Having her daughter in such a unit reassured her that everything that could be done was done, despite her daughter's ultimate death. She also saw the sense in consolidating diagnostic services in larger towns:

I don't think you miss out by living in the country. It's probably a bit harder with travelling and everything but in the last few years lots of things have come to the country that you used to have to go to the city for. The specialists are coming to major areas in the country, and the Magnetic Resonance scanners (MRI), and you no longer have to go to Sydney for your knee replacement. So I think they're waking up that it is more cost-effective to bring a lot out to a major spot in the country, bearing in mind that even our country areas are huge.

The stories I was told by patients in rural and remote areas were similar and rarely critical of their services despite their lack of access to specialist care. While geographical access was obviously a critical issue in times of emergency, the majority of people had realistic expectations of what can be delivered in an isolated community. And in such areas patient-driven models of care have emerged to meet the needs of the population and the context. Patient-driven models, which can be found in both rural and city areas, include women's health and community and primary care models.

H, who worked in the first Women's Health Centre in Australia, evaluated where this model was in today's contemporary climate of health care:

> While originally unencumbered with bureaucracy, women's
> health practices today have become part of Area Health Services
> along with the economic rhetoric and structures which in turn
> affect the practice, the language and therefore the culture. The
> newer nurses are therefore grafted onto the old model with its
> history since they were not part of the movement itself. But it is
> this history through which you learn your skills and knowledge
> about working with women.

Despite being under severe scrutiny in the current climate, the women's health model of care has been particularly resilient to political pressure, even triggering the demand for men's health centres that are being introduced in several states.

Community models of care are more inclusive of patients, and of the skills of each person in the community; they value sharing resources, being creative and using the resources at hand. Nurses and doctors working in such models generally have a much wider perspective of health, recognising the importance of public health strategies and education and employment as important determinants of well-being and quality of life. Some of this is driven by necessity since they do not have the resources available in large teaching hospitals where specialists in all disciplines abound. Instead, they become multiskilled and resourceful in tapping the community strengths.

W, an experienced nurse who has mainly worked in primary health care models, spoke of the advantages of community health models as 'looking at health before looking at illness and working with the community to manage all the things which are a major issue to the community'. This focus ensures that the needs that are met are those defined by patients rather than the professional.

Speaking of her experiences with Aboriginal health in isolated communities, W emphasised the role of opportunistic screening in such communities where it is less likely that individuals access routine facilities even if they are available. But while it seemed to be ideal she also noted the slowness of the model:

> If you take health care to the people, which is what the model is all about, you go to an Aboriginal community to see people who are sick but at the same time you say, 'Have you got an uncle in your family who is sick?' So you go and do TB screening. But I don't think it's that simple because some of the screening and tests you are providing are intrusive and so there needs to be time for people to take advantage of the health model of care.

The government driven models of care, such as hospital in the home and early discharge, are relatively new in terms of evaluation and critique, although nurses and doctors have expressed their concerns about the early discharge programs, particularly following complicated surgery. In the case of such models, while there is now clear evidence that hospitals are unsafe places in which to stay for long periods, there seems little doubt that the major driver is the need to cut the costs of hospitalisation. Both models of care do this by shifting costs, as well as the burden of care, to the patients and their families.

An expert stomal therapist spoke to me of her concerns over early discharge with the shortened length of stay for those who had stomas formed after surgery. Once she had days to prepare them for caring for their stoma when discharged, whereas now many go home not as well prepared given the length of time required by some to adapt to such a body image challenge. She overcomes this by following up patients when they come in for medical checkups and then later through the clinic attached to the ward. But many hospitals either do not provide follow up or do not have a person like H who breaks all the rules for the patients and is supported in doing so by the surgeons. Relying on individuals in the system is not an equitable or responsible way of managing care in a widespread and complex system, since this ultimately means that not all patients will have access to the best care. What we need are systems which work effectively for patients and for those working in the system. But what might such a system look like? John Wyn Owen, Executive Director of the Nuffield Health Trust in the UK, outlines the elements which contribute to the design of an ideal health system:

> The most successful health systems are those that have learned to get their strategy right. Planning, implementing and monitoring must be a never-ending process if it is to support growth and achieve satisfactory changes. Staff who work in the health service—doctors, nurses and other health professionals—are a key resource. There must be an appropriate level of investment in education and training to help people to do their jobs effectively and due recognition of excellence. The product of research development and a sense of critical evaluation of implementation must be integrated into all activities. Continual attention must be paid to attitudes and practice as well as access to data, information and intelligence with a focus on results and outcomes.[15]

7

—

Major challenges

In health we no longer work as a group in nursing, we now divide the care and you become specialised so you become isolated. You are not allowed to talk about the gall bladder if you are the breast cancer nurse. So if the breast cancer patient has a problem with their gall bladder then you need to hand over to the gall bladder specialist. (M)

I am utterly convinced that general medicine is an essential background to specialised medicine . . . The general physician should be able to think more broadly than the specialised person and yet he has to be able to think in almost the same depth that the specialised people do. There comes a time when you need to go to the super specialised person but the risk is that . . . the vast majority of people do not have single system disease. The interesting thing that is happening with Managed Care in the United States is that the general physician is coming back into his own and the managed care people have clear evidence that it is much more economical to use general physicians than a whole series of highly specialised ones. (J)

M, an experienced specialist nurse, and J, a Professor of Medicine and an eminent physician, separately spoke to me about the problems created by increased specialisation. They both highlighted the fragmentation faced not only by the patient but also by the professions. J also lamented the additional cost, overuse of certain technologies, and the lack of high level diagnostic skills which did not necessarily have to rely on invasive test results. Both of these highly skilled and experienced practitioners highlighted for me the contradictions inherent in our present health care system and the difficulties in managing health care in our contemporary society—a society which makes more demands of a system which needs massive restructuring if it is to be relevant.

H, a pensioner, highlighted the need for integration of the various sectors of the system when she spoke of her concerns about the division between the public and private and the state and federal sectors:

> Communication is needed urgently between health service and community service. There's not enough communication between doctors and GPs and their patients and between services. There's no communication between doctors and nursing homes and this needs to be explored further.

So many patients spoke to me about going home from hospital and then having to ring their general practitioner and explain what had happened to them in hospital. Despite discharge summaries being part of the routine in hospital (on paper) so often they did not reach the general practitioner who had to follow up the management of the patient. This is but one part of any new model of care we adopt. It needs to be designed to overcome the present fragmentation of care, lack of individual attention and awareness of specific needs, lack of access to expertise and facilities, and increasing costs, which many of the patients' stories in this book have already illustrated. Each one of these problems has sub-categories, such as the increasing specialisation which not only adds costs to the system but means that patients feel that no one is viewing them as a whole. In turn this increases the feelings of alienation and lack of individual attention. It also creates division between the professionals working in the various specialities.

Alternative models to ensure a better integration of care are urgently required given the shortened length of hospital stay for patients, the complex nature of treatments and drug therapy, the emerging fragmentation of the system and the shifting of responsibility to the consumer. While the models of care discussed previously may have their place in our changing system, in the main they have developed piecemeal with limited evaluation or analysis of their place in the total system of care. Not that we are alone in our dilemma—it is an international one with New Zealand, Canada, the UK and the USA all attempting to reconfigure their systems over the last decade.

INTERNATIONAL MODELS

Some attempts at remodelling health care, such as UK Prime Minister Tony Blair's 'third way', have been more radical than others, and remain untested. The USA has continued with a privatised system despite its obvious inequalities and economic contradictions.

The Canadian health care system, which is perhaps most like ours in many ways, is substantially a one-class system. It is administered by the provinces according to need and guided by the principles of Medicare: universality, comprehensive coverage of 'medically necessary' services, inter-provincial portability, not-for-profit operation, and with a prohibition on out-of-pocket patient charges. This devolution of administrative and fiscal responsibility avoids the complex state/federal system we have in Australia, which contributes to problems associated with cost-shifting. It may also encourage a wider population-based approach to resource distribution and care. In the Canadian model, doctors' fees are capped at both individual and speciality level in consultation with provincial medical associations. As a direct result, hospital admissions have been reduced. And despite the prohibition on up-front patient charges and the not-for-profit ethos removing financial competition from the system, between 1998 and 1999 Canada reduced its health expenditure from 10 per cent to 9 per cent of gross domestic product, at the same time as ours rose from 7.7 per cent to 8.4 per cent. This directly challenges the notion that competition in health reduces costs. However, Deeble notes one major gap in Canadian health care and that is in the lack of a Pharmaceutical Benefits Scheme (PBS) which means that out of hospital drugs are far more expensive than in Australia,[1] a major concern given the importance of drug regimes to so many people with chronic illnesses.

110

Delivering an effective and efficient system which meets individual and population health needs seems an almost impossible ask given our complex system, yet it is a complexity which Canada has gone a long way to overcome. A Canadian health care professional, C, who had been working in Australia for a year, spoke to me about her attempts to negotiate the minefield of the Australian health care system:

> I'm still having trouble figuring out how Australian health care private and public systems work together. I don't know whether they interface or whether they work in parallel or whether they in fact work in competition but certainly in my personal experience in having to have orthopaedic surgery here there seems to be no options to get an arthroscopy in any other way except your private care. And if I was to go to a public clinic I was told that I would be waiting for two years. Well I couldn't walk so I couldn't wait for two years.
>
> Now in Canada with our universal health care system, each of the doctors has a billing number and I would choose whatever doctor I want to go to and I would be referred to a specialist but I would still have a choice of them. The other thing that is important is that our doctors earn whatever they can through the billing to Medicare since fees are capped, unlike here.

MODELS IN PROGRESS

Case management is one model of care that has the potential to meet the challenges inherent in our contemporary health care system. While it has been used in other sectors, such as social security and mental health, it is a recent introduction to acute health care services. As M explains: 'As a Case Manager I see the patient in the pre-admission clinic or the doctor's rooms after diagnosis. I follow them up in a week to prepare them for surgery.' M, an experienced nurse, continued to talk to me about her role as a Case Manager with women diagnosed with breast cancer and undergoing surgery. She spoke of enrolling in an advanced counselling course to help her with her role since:

A lot of my time is taken up with counselling. I also work out if their partner needs counselling and I liaise with other professionals. I then see the patient in the hospital but only about once since I don't want to take over from the nurses [in the hospital]. Then I follow them up in the clinic and during chemotherapy to support them. I sometimes do a home visit but I really don't have time.

Case management is being implemented successfully across many areas of illness care, such as cardiothoracic surgery, breast cancer and chronic respiratory disease, throughout Australia. The Case Manager becomes the pivotal practitioner in the continuum of care involving education and support of patient, family and friends, ensuring that the care is always appropriate and safe, and sensitive to the needs of the patient. As M comments:

I work in a medical team but from the nurse's point of view the advantage is to have a better picture of the patient and their prognosis for counselling and to understand the different doctors' practices and likes and dislikes.

Case management is rated highly by patients but is certainly labour intensive, with even a devoted nurse like M claiming that she feels burnt out, giving herself five years in the role. M believes that 'It was badly introduced across the medical system since the doctors were suspicious that the nurse was going to "manage" them'. She works very long hours with no additional salary or benefits, carries a pager and supplies her own car. Presently on leave, she was concerned that she had no replacement so the women undergoing surgery while she was away did not have a Case Manager. M believes that, in the future, the Case Manager should work more across the community, liaising with the general practitioners who are increasingly being identified as the coordinators of care for women with breast cancer, a move M supports wholeheartedly.

Case management is a model similar to that used by the palliative care nurse who works across an Area Health Service following patients between home and hospital as required, and liaising with doctors and allied health professionals. In many cases the palliative care nurse also ensures that the patient can die at home by her being there until the end with the family. In this way the nurse manages the case (that is, the patient's episode of care).

Patient-focused models of care such as case management are ideal in terms of overcoming the limitations of our fragmented system and in facilitating communication across sectors. They ensure that the patient's needs are central to the care given, that all the necessary information is transferred, that the patient feels safe and informed, and that support is in place whether that be in hospital, a nursing home or at home. The positive responses from patients and families to case management are not only validating its worth to patient outcomes, but are also affirming the worth of the nurse who practices in such a model of care. The nurses I spoke to who work as Case Managers receive enormous professional satisfaction because of the patient-centred nature of the model. Such staff satisfaction is rare in today's health care arena and is to be encouraged in order to retain experienced nurses, many of whom are leaving the system.[2] Labour-intensive and requiring experienced and highly skilled staff, such models, however, are not necessarily attractive to those who hold the purse strings. Policy makers whose planning is often based on short-term economic strategies may not recognise how cost-effective Case Managers are, if only in the area of preventing adverse events, readmission and post-operative complications.

The Nurse Practitioner is another emerging model of care in rural and remote areas in NSW and in other contexts in several other states. This model has only recently been legislated for in NSW after ten years of struggle by nurses. In many cases it is a validation of the role nurses are already playing in the remote areas of Australia in that they are practising an extended role well beyond the traditional role of the nurse. They often work alone with no medical or other nursing or allied health support. They are on call 24 hours a day yet are often paid at the lowest end of the nursing salary. M exemplifies the typical nurse working in an isolated rural town with limited support.

> You wouldn't think that in the morning I'm seeing Aboriginal babies and in the afternoon I'm doing a Guardianship Board

hearing and that night I'm in a police car going to put someone in hospital. I do pub crawls to find my clients because they need an injection. With the ones I am treating for a long time I just go in and say 'your needle's due'. They know their needle's due but they've got no money to pay for their script so I've bought their script. I do it because it's the weekend and I know that if they 'go off' I'll spend three hours in the back of an ambulance with them escorting them to X. I've recently had to escort three scheduled patients because there is no one else to go. Usually they pay the money back.

M earns $30 000 annually, is a registered nurse and midwife, an experienced palliative care and early childhood nurse and also works within the nearby Aboriginal community as often as she can since they have no Aboriginal nurse.

The implementation of the Nurse Practitioner role will enable many nurses such as M to apply for authorisation but they will only be employed in such a role if it is advertised in their area and they are successful in their application for the position. The initial Nurse Practitioner roles will be established and advertised in those areas which have been identified by all stakeholders as 'areas of need'. The authorisation process which is a separate process has been set up by a multidisciplinary group under the direction of the Nurses Registration Board. This process involves each applicant putting together an extensive portfolio of academic and practical experience with proof of high quality care and outcomes followed by an oral examination for those whose portfolios reflect the necessary standard.

The Nurse Practitioner model offers many advantages. In rural or remote communities the Nurse Practitioner takes a population/community perspective as well as being able to manage emergency situations, wound dressing, post-natal care, early discharge from hospital, the mentally and physically disabled, and the frail elderly who may need supervision if they are remaining in their own home, which is so often the case in a small community. Immunisation clinics and baby health care centres are also conducted by nurses in these areas at the same time as they are educating the community about healthy living. S, a community nurse in an isolated rural community, has also received a grant to run a local picture show while J obtained computers for literacy classes. It is envisaged that, despite ongoing concerns being expressed by the Australian Medical Association (AMA), the Nurse Practitioners will also provide support for doctors working in isolated practices in terms of referral, ordering medications and interpreting results. They will work as colleagues in the interests of the patient to ensure more efficient and certainly cost-effective and appropriate management. Already evaluation of the early Nurse Practitioner model is being established and there has been widespread community support for this model of care.

Managed care,[3] a model of funding which is transforming the design and delivery of health care in the USA, is currently under review here. Health Management Organisations (HMOs) through managed care have an increasing monopoly on health care insurance in the USA, providing health care at a predetermined cost while at the same time restricting the type of care and the context in which that care can be received—that is, the hospital and the provider. While this model has been shown to cut costs in the USA, it remains problematic because of the many case studies which demonstrate its mismanagement at all levels—particularly when it comes to the emergency situation. Poor outcomes, inefficient services and inequities in terms of access for those most in need have increased the gap between the rich and poor in health despite a thriving economy. The USA not only has poorer health outcomes than Australia, it also has groups with no or only limited access to health care.

As a result of this discontent with the system in the USA there is considerable change underway, necessitated by marketplace economics rather than by the federal government, which failed in its efforts to reform health care under President Clinton. The main drivers of the change are: the buyers of health care, which are the employers in most cases; the patients, who find the system so complicated to use; the increased cost of technology; and the demographics of the country, where so many people still have no access to health care and health improvement strategies have been neglected.

Richard Davidson, president of the American Hospitals Association, speaks about the move for health plans in some states to collaborate on the very expensive services, such as community-wide ventures in health improvement strategies, while remaining as competitors in delivering acute services. This way they are able to offer broader health plans to employers. As Richardson said, 'We think that if we are going to have a competitive model play itself out and be effective then that is what is going to happen. You are going to have to find ways to reconcile these differences.'[4] As a result of this, many hospitals are changing their models of care by taking care into the workplace, schools and community, providing a continuum of care rather than just acute services.

While Australian medical groups have rejected managed care in any form, it remains a potential approach in this country, supported in a modified form by the present Federal Minister for Health who criticises the previous Labor government's limited view of the private system as 'monocular'. Dr Michael Wooldridge, the Minister for Health in a government that has embraced marketplace principles and privatisation, claims the private hospital system is 'an essential ingredient in the nation's health care'.[5] In his 1997 proposed legislative amendments to sustain the private sector, Wooldridge built in a more attractive scheme for contracting between insurance funds, hospitals and doctors. By enabling the health benefit funds to pay benefits above the Medical Benefits Schedule to specific doctors who qualify, out-of-pocket costs for patients should be either excluded or at least known before the event. Given the disillusionment expressed by patients about the lack of certainty with the costs of services, this was intended to encourage a return to private insurance.

Given that our system has followed, but is not as radical (or as cost-efficient) as, the National Health System (NHS) in the UK, and given that even Wooldridge acknowledges that 'Australians overwhelmingly support Medicare and the universal access to public health services that this entails',[6] perhaps the NHS has something to offer. After all the NHS has been through the era of market forces in the 1990s in which general practitioners could be both providers of health and, through the granting of an annual budget, purchasers of health care services including emergency services.

The NHS model was adopted with modifications in 1992 in New Zealand, which subsequently experienced the same early problems and obstacles as the NHS. These included the fact that competition and market forces were not necessarily appropriate or effective in health care where collaboration is essential and rationing difficult to determine or mandate. There was no incentive to share knowledge or expertise, and inequities occurred when certain practitioners were able to obtain better services than others, and unprofitable patients were not serviced adequately. And, unlike other marketplaces, it has been shown that the demand for health care is not necessarily contained by increasing the cost of the product to the consumer (see Donaldson's critique of this below).

The integrated model of care is the new UK framework introduced in 1997. Prime Minister Tony Blair calls this 'the third way' which is 'based on partnership and driven by performance'.[7] The latter will be measured not solely by crude economic indicators but also by health outcomes. Perhaps the most radical element of this new model is the Health Improvement Programs which acknowledge all determinants of health by encouraging integration between health services and social services, housing, education and employment. Primary care groups consisting of general practitioners, community nurses and primary care staff will also be part of this model, as will multidisciplinary teams. This model seems most appropriate for Australia given our current weaknesses, and the lack of integration across sectors that undoubtedly determine health status—housing, social security, employment and education.

WEIGHING THE ALTERNATIVES

There is no doubt that the major problem we are facing today is how to meet all the demands on our system without an increase in the budget. At the present time it could be said that the fact that our system is still largely publicly funded is one of the most positive aspects of our health care. It does mean that, in the main, everyone has access to a certain level of health care when they need it. Of course, the reality is that this may be only after waiting for transport, travelling long distances, and waiting for medical help, which may not then be culturally sensitive.

But the key issue here is that no one is denied health care in Australia in the twenty-first century and certainly we have extremely efficient emergency medical care systems and high quality professional staff. Compared with the millions who presently do not have access to health care in the USA, let alone the billions in less developed countries, we have a highly effective system of health care.

The major concern we presently face, therefore, is whether we can continue with such a quality system without increasing the amount spent on health care by governments. In the next few years funding will be the key issue underpinning changes to our health care and already there are signs that we are moving away from a fully publicly funded system to one which shifts costs to the patients. Concern about this trend was fuelled in 1998 by the federal government offering a 30 per cent rebate to those taking out private health insurance in an effort to decrease those abandoning the private system while boosting the numbers of those joining it. Present trends also reflect a move towards users paying more for the care they receive at the point of contact.

Lifetime Health Cover was also introduced in 2000, not as a carrot but as a stick approach to persuade individuals into taking out private insurance. This penalty scheme enforces higher premiums for individuals who delay joining a health insurance fund after 30 years of age and as a result of this and the 30 per cent rebate, an additional two million have joined private health insurance funds. This increase is cited as evidence of success in reducing the strain on public hospitals but given that such an increase means reduced funding to the public system and that despite being privately insured we are all entitled to access the public system through our Medicare contribution, it is spurious evidence.[8] Indeed the federal government's Productivity Commission found that given most people receiving the rebate are already insured there will be little additional impact on the public system. They also found that even privately insured patients still use the public system during emergencies and complicated surgical procedures which involve high medical co-payments.[9]

Professor Steven Duickett, who is former head of the Commonwealth Department of Health, was also critical of these government 'incentives': 'The 30 per cent (health insurance) rebate is effectively a subsidy to the private health insurance industry and is larger than the budgetary assistance for the mining, manufacturing and primary agricultural industries combined.'[10]

Given the indirect shift to 'user pays' in parts of our system, any new model of management which we might choose may also bring with it an up-front fee. For example, case management could be perceived merely as an added cost to a service and even one which users should pay for. The same could happen with any service outside acute care, given our illness-driven system. This would erode choice and equity leaving us with a system that creates even greater division between the rich and the poor. It would thus negate the advances we have made, such as the move to involving patients in their care and designing services to indi-vidualise care.

The current reality is that we have an increasingly pressured public system that does not always deliver the best care to all because of increased turnover of patients who are more frail and compromised. R, a patient, in discussing the obvious shortage of staff during her hospitalisation, told her story of a nurse who continually said she didn't have time or she had to catch a bus. R said all that she expects from a nurse or doctor is:

> . . . to get the feeling that they are not overworked and that looking after me is of prime importance to them even if they have a million things to do. I'm not demanding, but when they're with me I expect them to be focused on me and my needs.

R speaks for every patient I have spoken with, as far as wanting to feel that the nurse and doctor are paying attention to their individual needs.

So, how can we deliver this individualised care which, after all, seems the least patients should expect and should have? Is a user pays model the answer? It is after all, not without a well-established and argued ideology which makes sense to many as an attractive alternative. Specifically, it is based on the belief that any government-aided system has 'the tendency to develop a psy-chology of dependence and diminished personal and community responsibility'.[11] While once confined to the conservative side of politics, this belief now appears to pervade the entire political spectrum, emerging in other sectors previously fully supported by government funding, such as education and social security. While there is no doubt that education and social security are vital to a society, and even to the health of a society, health care has an additional urgency factor because of the potential for premature death to occur in cases where care is not available. And while this occasionally happens today it is certainly not routine. A situation where individuals are unable to access care if it had to be paid for up-front is something we should avoid at all costs.

Sharing resources equitably across a country such as Australia with its geographical limitations in terms of access is also part of the funding debate. To confound this we already have a history of massive political shifts in resource distribution. The Whitlam era, with its vision of a welfare state uniting many entities in an attempt to gain a more total approach to health, contrasts with the present conservative era of the commodification of health. Commodification is justified by governments as they face the rising cost of health. It is the same argument or justification employed by other public corporations such as education and social security.

But these ideological shifts have not occurred in a vacuum. A multiplicity of global changes accompanied or even preceded them, not the least of which is the move to managerialism as the 'new' way to efficient and effective organisation of both public and private organisations. And accompanying managerialism is the latest business ideology such as competitive markets, benchmarking and restructuring, all relatively foreign to health in the past and still untested in terms of advantage to the health of our nation.

Ironically, the consumer movement itself may have been inadvertently implicated in this shift away from government responsibility because of its challenge to the traditional, paternalistic model of care. While apparently well meant, the traditional beneficence model in health relied on an expert group determining the health needs of society and was thus perceived to have disempowered individuals and communities. However, while the consumer's claim to shared power is to be celebrated, it also assists the shift to user pays since it can be argued that patients are now educated enough to look after their own health, and to take responsibility for their own management of illness and that of others. Of course, such a generalisation is flawed in its assumption that individuals are equally well educated and informed, that they are in supportive social units, and that they are employed and have the resources to access health care as they require it. The patients' stories in this book reveal wide differences in the ability to pay, to manage alone, or to support others.

Take, for example, the woman who spoke of her inability to contact anyone because of the STD block on her phone due to her straitened financial situation. This only compounds her problem of gaining access to help with a health problem. She is already disadvantaged by geographical isolation. Her financial status means that she lives from day-to-day, relying on social security payments. She lives in a rural area with a very high unemployment rate so, even if she had the skills and access, would be very unlikely to gain employment.

The introduction of a user pays system might not cause her additional hardship directly if she was entitled to free health care (which cannot be assured), but she may suffer indirect discrimination because of her financial and social status. She would very likely be required to wait longer for service and for surgery if the latest trend analysis concerning waiting times for public versus private patients is to be believed. And if this trend moved even further toward a fully privatised system then we have the American experience to warn us of the massive inequities in such a system.

Apparently unconcerned by such warnings, our present federal government recently flagged a move to ask non-government agencies to tender for the care of the developmentally disabled, thus abdicating their responsibility to the most disempowered group of all. This group includes women like Amanda who is autistic, deaf, and unable to speak, suffering at the hands of untrained carers who failed to treat her medical problems, causing her to become frustrated and violent.[12] When Amanda began head butting the walls the police were called; they handcuffed her, wrapped her in a sheet, and put her in the back of a paddy wagon.

Recent debates have also raised the issue of up-front payments for health care in hospitals at the point of contact. While our present system may suffer from inequities, at least access is not dependent on being able to pay. Of course, we already have a user pays system according to financial ability through mandatory taxation; this is an extremely equitable system and is not as publicly obvious as an up-front payment. I observed the processing of up-front payments in an American hospital emergency department and a certain discrimination as those holding Medicaid cards were stood to one side while those paying up-front were placed on the waiting list. It was a form of public humiliation that leads to those needing health care the most avoiding it in order to avoid discrimination.

Cam Donaldson, from the UK Institute for Public Policy Research, claims 'charges have a greater impact on those in lower income groups and that this may have possible adverse effects on their health'.[13] This impact is caused by many factors as an empirical study of dental care in the UK showed.[14] In this study those who paid an up-front fee (the non-exempt) were 340 times more likely to get a check up than those who were exempt because of financial difficulties. The latter group received 40 per cent less treatment than the non-exempt group. This was not about individuals accessing care but about professional accountability to those who are unable to pay for services and who are subsidised by the government. While this study was undertaken in the UK, it nevertheless raises questions about possible indirect discrimination by service providers which is often disguised and revealed only through research such as this.

Donaldson also argues that while added cost will usually reduce consumption of a product, evidence from the USA shows that rather than decreasing when costs rise, health consumption increases. He puts this down to the fact that doctors have an incentive to maintain incomes, as does any profession; thus even if demand from one group, such as the poor, reduces when costs rise, services increase for other groups who can afford the charges. Consumption, and therefore costs, of health care are not reduced but shifted across groups causing the World Health Organization to condemn the practice of user pays in health as inequitable:[15]

> Health systems world-wide have failed to recognise the
> implications of the fundamental shift in the paradigm that has
> come to dominate economic and social development over the

last decade. The paradigm can be paraphrased as 'the market approach'. It poses a number of fundamental challenges to the pursuit of health for all. These include the advancement of the notion that health is merely a commodity and, as such, has a price and can be traded off against other commodities. [What is needed] is a radical reorientation towards development of health systems whose goal is the improvement of the health status and well being of entire populations with priority to those in greatest need.[16]

This condemnation of the privileging of economic efficiency over and above social equity in this WHO report flags a warning to those countries, including Australia, which have adopted such a value system. Not that economic efficiency is unimportant in an environment where costs are increasing and demands are rising, but equity deserves close scrutiny and action when health status and access inequities are as evident as they are in Australia today. This means that the economic efficiencies have to be made in the appropriate places to ensure a system of delivery balance which best meets the needs of as many Australians as possible.

Pensioners are one of the groups feeling most vulnerable in the Australian system, with the obvious shift towards user pays. They perceive that present governments undervalue the worth of the elderly. As B told me:

> When I was expressing my concern about closing down my hospital and when I said, 'Who would I get to look after me if I were sick?' my doctor, who is much younger than me of course, said 'Well, you've got your family'. So this is the attitude, you're getting older now, we don't treat too many people after they're 70, we don't bother with them very much . . . Older people aren't being treated properly now.

While figures from acute hospitals do not support this, the issue here is the perception of the Pensioners and Superannuants consumer group I interviewed. It was a perception backed by many personal experiences of the group in their interactions with the health system.

Key challenges

The key challenges facing the Australian health care system flow from the failure of conventional health care systems around the developed world to anticipate the massive social, political and economic changes which would sweep the developed world in the final decades of the twentieth century. The impact of economic rationalism in the 1980s, which valorised the application of contemporary business principles and practice in health, education and social welfare, offered governments a philosophical justification for abandoning their conventional responsibilities to fund the public sector. Yet, while governments have justified this move on the grounds of efficiency as costs rise across all these sectors, they have often failed to identify the structural problems within these systems which are driving costs up.

In the Australian health care sector the trend of increased costs has, in fact, been largely driven by the culture of the system itself, a system that has emerged with minimal restrictions. The main drivers have been increased use of expensive technology, medical advances and the structure of medical payments in parallel with an increased education of and demand by consumers, an ageing population and, consequently, a higher turnover of patients through the acute sector.

Despite the fact that the payment structure for visiting medical officers in public hospitals actually provides a built-in incentive to increase medical services, patients are still blamed for the increase in demand without a more rigorous critique of the whole equation of supply and demand. Patients are certainly paying for such demand through reduced access to or reduced quality of services, or through increased costs. The question of how many services are inappropriate, that is, those being delivered without good evidence that the outcomes are beneficial to the patient, is also an emerging issue and a costly one. Measuring inappropriate services is difficult, however evidence is emerging when comparing public and private practices that there is an increased rate of medical intervention in the private sector following heart attack[17] as well as a higher rate of birth by caesarian section in the private sector.[18] Neither of these rates can be explained through extraneous variables such as socioeconomic or co-morbidities. The system therefore requires not only an analysis of use but also of misuse and abuse, much of which is not transparent.

While the official rhetoric about health directions in Australia —for example, the NSW Health Strategic Directions for Health 1998–2003; *Better Health, Good Health Care*—suggests that a radical reorientation has already been embraced, the major efforts appear to be put into hospitals and illness care rather than into primary health care strategies or community-based programs.

It seems, therefore, that the reality on the ground is very different—as the stories in this book attest. Of course, individual stories may be dismissed as unrepresentative, but in a system that prides itself on being up there with the best internationally, there are far too many stories which defy this self-assured image.

Given the world-wide evidence and high level advice against moving towards a more user pays system, and given that Australia, compared to many other countries, delivers a very high standard of care in a cost-effective manner, the question becomes: to what degree should we attempt to change the current system? We know where the increased costs are in the system, we know which groups have poorer health status, we know the inequities in the system. Where do we begin, given the failure of successive Australian governments attempting health care reform in the past?[19]

8

—

Future delivery of care

> One man from Mudgee in NSW described how all the medical centres in the town had refused to bulk bill and how his wife had been turned away for a regular prescription for heart medicine because she could not pay for the consultation even though she offered to pay on the next pension day.[1]

Chris Sidoti, lawyer and human rights activist, reflected on this story as he spoke of the Human Rights Commission's consultancy in regional, rural and remote Australia. Merrilyn Walton, ex-Health Care Complaints Commissioner in NSW, recently spoke of the record number of complaints by patients about the way they are treated by nurses and doctors, including allegations of rudeness, carelessness, incompetence and unethical conduct.[2] And, as I have already outlined in Chapter 5, the socially and economically disadvantaged continue to face problems accessing adequate health care even in our present system. Sidoti identified Indigenous people, older people and those younger people who required access to mental health expertise as most disadvantaged in the rural areas he visited. He found that many indigenous people would rather die than leave family, community and land to gain access to care such as renal dialysis outside their community, while the elderly are often forced to seek an aged care facility outside the community where they have always lived, thus 'leaving town to die'.[3] And as for the young, 'the community sees children as problems to be endured not our future to be nurtured'.[4]

Of course, as I've noted throughout this book, it would be unrealistic to expect our system to be flawless given its complex financial and administrative structures. Such structures produce dependence on a mixture of state and federal politics, transitory strategic planning because of triennial changes in governments, fragmentation through geographic, disciplinary and contextual boundaries and interests, and an intransigent culture which avoids social and cultural change. But it is equally unrealistic and unethical to ignore the challenge of what we have created—an intervention treadmill of demand and supply which is never-ending. And we have done so at the expense of other priority areas. Health care has become synonymous with hospital care, which translates into illness care. Perhaps it has always been this way because of our cultural understandings of what a health care system is designed to do, but we now have evidence which challenges such traditional notions.

Today we know where the most urgent problems lie and what they are; where health care delivery is inadequate; what consumers want; and where fragmentation and, therefore lack of continuity of care occurs. The time is right for us to demand a system that is truly about the health of society, not only its illness. This requires hard decisions about reconfiguring our narrow illness-focused health care system to one that is inclusive of all the population, understanding the contexts in which they live and get sick, and acknowledging their differences and their priorities. It will also demand a shifting of resources, human and fiscal. It does not necessarily mean building more hospitals, but rather planning appropriate models of health care better tailored to the needs of specific groups and contexts.

MANAGING RESOURCES

What to fund and what not to fund is a daily concern at all levels of the health care system, but the broader question of resource distribution is rarely debated at any length. Every day we read of the desperate plight of the health care sector in terms of Area Health Services that are debt-ridden, waiting lists that are growing, and hospitals being closed. It seems that at every meeting I attend, funding raises its ugly head, but no longer does it even raise a collective sigh, suggesting battle fatigue. It is as if the mantra is 'it needs to be this way' rather than 'why is it this way?' In relation to health care, the solution becomes quite simple to those whose role is to balance the budget but not give the care—cut all the things on the red side of the ledger: namely, nursing and cleaning staff. Immediately, the budget becomes healthier. Meanwhile, what about the health of the patients?

A recent example answers this question, an example that headed the news for several weeks.[5] It involved the use of kerosene baths for treating scabies in a nursing home. The consequence of this action was the burning of the skin of many of the elderly residents. Such a short-term, old-fashioned, cost-cutting measure to treat a widespread hygiene problem was not only barbaric, it was economically inefficient in terms of long-term outcomes, and experienced and educated nursing staff would have given that advice. Adequate cleaning staff may even have prevented the infection from occurring. In other words, economic efficiency and good patient care are not necessarily mutually exclusive. In fact, many preventive strategies often have long-term economic benefits but so often there are short-term directives requiring answers. And given that the effectiveness of a service today is so often measured in terms of coming in on budget, it is understandable that decisions will not necessarily be based on what is best for the patient if that might cost more.

Compounding this particular case is the increasing privatisation of care of the elderly in this country. As caring for the aged has become identified as a new niche market in which to invest, it is little wonder that incidents like the above occur. And if this is so, then it is difficult to accuse proprietors of nursing homes who conduct their businesses in ways which make a profit. After all, the move to privatise aged care was a political one underpinned by legislative change which controlled subsidies to nursing homes. The 1997 *Residential Aged Care Act* brought in by the present federal government has meant that no longer is there a targeted amount specifically to be used for personal care as there was in the past. This means that it is up to the managers and/or the proprietors to decide where the subsidies are spent, on the residents or elsewhere.

While cost containment has been the main driver in many areas of health, particularly in the last two decades, some sectors appear to have been corralled from the need to argue for their funding. This has been compounded by the lack of local and national debate with consumers and health care workers about how and why resources are distributed. Hence a system in continual crisis. Funds never match the needs of what will continue to be a bottomless pit of demand and service if we don't make some hard decisions. After all, when their health is threatened, most people want a cure and will go to enormous lengths to obtain one. When professionals want new equipment, new structures or new staff, the arguments are equally compelling.

The argument about how much is enough should not be held at the bedside of the patient, but out in the community in a series of well-informed debates to avoid difficult and even unethical decision-making on the spot, as so often is the case. We all have a responsibility to decide how much we are prepared to spend on health or illness, knowing that it may mean less funding for education or transport, or less available income for many of us if the public consensus is to fund increased services through increases in taxation. Community-wide consultation would be a more transparent and fairer way to manage resource distribution since, along with the consumer, those managing health in community programs, working in primary health care teams or in the aged and disability sectors, are so often left out of the main debates about resource distribution.

Another solution to the rising costs and one gaining momentum is to extend privatisation and there are sections of the community and the professions who believe this is the answer to the funding crisis. That is, they view health care like any commodity—it should be bought by the individual. However, as I have argued previously in this book, the health of individuals is not like other commodities in that it is so often not about choosing to be ill or not to be ill. As Professor Stephen Leeder, Dean of Medicine at the University of Sydney, in addressing the ethics of resource distribution in health, comments:

> We know little about the distribution of health-care resources [in Australia today] and just a bit more about the way in which health is distributed. The health of Australians has improved dramatically in the last century and continues to improve . . . yet health is not distributed equitably. The capricious randomness with

which one person develops cancer, another has a heart attack and so on is exacerbated by the persistent and disturbing themes of maldistribution of health that are present in our community.[6]

Illness certainly touches everyone in some way in their lifetime, regardless of socioeconomic circumstance. But we do know that environments—social, economic and cultural—play a vital part in one's health.[7] How, then, do we justify the discrimination that occurs if we demand that everyone pays up-front for health care? While proponents of the user pays model claim that disadvantaged groups would continue to have free care, there is always a proportion of the population not eligible for financial support but who are nevertheless economically disadvantaged who will find it difficult to pay up-front and will simply not be able to access adequate care.

The above arguments do not, of course, preclude having a private sector within the public system for those who can afford and choose to pay for the additional comforts or advantages, such as shorter waiting times or a single room. This has been the case for some time now and will likely continue to be so, whatever changes are made. It is even arguable that a well-managed private sector might take some of the present pressure off the public system if it were well supported. As medical insurance groups continue to negotiate 'no gap' insurance deals with hospitals and doctors, the percentage who take up private insurance may increase to ensure a more viable private system. But we need always to keep in mind the potential inequities of privatisation.

C spoke to me about one such inequity she encountered having to wait weeks for an MRI in a public hospital, which she could have accessed privately that same day:

> If you're a person who has maybe a brain tumour or something wrong with your spine, the offer that for $1000 you can come in tomorrow and get the diagnosis, but you may have to wait for two weeks in the public system, is not a choice for those without the $1000 and even for those who have $1000.

And D, a public patient in the Australian system who spoke to me of her recent spinal surgery, had no wait for an MRI but a two-week wait for surgery:

I'd already been through three months of pain so I felt that it wasn't a 'surgery at all costs' idea. Then when I made the decision it was very quick . . . he [the neurosurgeon] said 'We can do it in a fortnight's time'.

DE, on the other hand, chose not to wait several weeks for a public bed following the discovery of a brain tumour on an MRI scan. 'I just wanted to get rid of it', she said. She was admitted within 24 hours but she needed to go to a private hospital. As she told me she was 'one of the lucky ones who could afford private health care'.

In the 1960s, private health care was also there for those who chose to access it but choice was far more narrow because of the relative lack of sophisticated technological procedures. Choice was therefore limited to the doctor and the hospital, although these were restricted in most cases to availability. Choice of closed or open surgery, of epidural pain relief or caesarean section for birth, of day surgery, of home dialysis, of one drug over another for the same disorder, of early discharge, were not even on the agenda. Today, choice is both everywhere and nowhere. It can be overwhelming for those who live in large cities and are economically viable and educated, as well as those who are privately insured. It is often not the case for those in remote and even some rural areas without access, certainly not for those who are unable to pay or understand their rights, and even at times for anyone who lives at great distances from available health care.

So how do we manage increasing demand and neglected needs along with individual choice and increasing costs in a political environment which has until now been driven by a marketplace mentality?

SIGNS OF REFORM

It seems that there is a shift occurring in terms of governments acknowledging the need to find solutions which are compatible with the ideologies of informed and politically sensitive lobby groups such as those in rural areas. State and federal governments, along with consumers and professionals, are initiating structural reforms not necessarily reliant on the privatisation solution. One example is the NSW Health Council whose report has just been released recommending new models of care delivery to overcome fragmentation, ensure better continuity of care, address the needs of the chronically ill and balance the inequities within rural and remote communities. John Menadue, the Chairman of the Health Council, distilled some of the essence of the report in his message at the beginning of the report:

> In the course of our work, I often speculated that we should have been called the Hospital Council. So much of our work and so much of the 'health debate' is really about hospitals and sickness rather than health. The desire of many clinicians and managers to shift resources and provide more care in the community with an increased emphasis on both early intervention and keeping people well, gets lost in the clamour for more beds and more expensive facilities in hospitals.[8]

Recent federal government initiatives are also attempting to address some of the current inequities that have already meant a change in resource distribution through incentive payments to general practitioners who play a key role in primary health care.

These incentives are central to the federal government's Enhanced Primary Care Package (EPCP) presently being implemented in each state with funding already allocated in the federal budget. The EPCP certainly places an increased emphasis on the role of the general practitioner looking after a population through improved coordination between general practitioners and others involved in primary health care teams; improved information to consumers and health professionals; voluntary health assessments for people aged 75 years or over; and care planning and case conferencing for people with chronic and complex health care needs. This is being funded through the Medical Benefits Schedule, thus providing incentives for general practitioners to work in these new models. It is underpinned by improved electronic data interchange, widespread education of general practitioners and consumers and the establishment of standards and guidelines by the Royal Australian College of General Practitioners (RACGP).

Another harbinger of change is the National Public Health

Partnership (NPHP) which is attempting to integrate approaches to chronic disease prevention. As Dr Andrew Wilson, the chair of NPHP, puts it:

> This provides an opportunity for the Partnership to link with the work of the National Health Priority Areas initiative offering a strong holistic prevention component on a cluster of conditions which integrates national action on priority areas . . . providing a more appropriate focus that moves away from 'body parts', builds on extensive planning already undertaken and understandable to clinicians, decision makers and consumers.[9]

National Health Priority Areas include cardiovascular health, cancer control, injury prevention and control, mental health and diabetes mellitus and, more recently, asthma, most of which are identified as chronic illnesses which add to the burden of disease in this country, and certainly are major problems in certain Indigenous and rural populations. But whatever the category, the important issue is the impact each of these events or illnesses has on the lives of individuals and their families. Certainly in terms of costs, prevention is the cheaper alternative, recognised and acknowledged but rarely funded with resources at the same level as those applied to acute illnesses and surgical intervention—intervention which does not necessarily correct the underlying chronic disease such as in the case of cardiac or widespread vascular disease.

SHIFTING OUR FOCUS

Despite these signs of change, as far as actually implementing structural reform in Australia we have remained relatively timid, merely working around the edges. Such timidity can be explained away on the basis of vested interests determining the agenda, as Sax has proposed in his *Strife of Interests*.[10] Not that understanding the obstacles to reform necessarily helps those who work in the system or those who are at the end of the production line—the patients. We need to be more courageous if we are to reorient a system whose culture and structures remain inflexible and which do not meet the needs of so many populations. We need to say 'enough is enough' in some areas and redistribute resources, or agree that we want everything and are prepared to pay for it.

Any decision, of course, demands a change in approach not only on the part of professionals, politicians, researchers and policy makers, but also consumers. If we act on the knowledge that, for example, attention to lifestyle, improved drugs and surgery have all contributed to the 60 per cent decline in the death rate from heart disease since the 1960s,[11] then it seems clear what our focus needs to be. After all, we are a culture which has a widespread reliance on surgery or drugs to cure. And while in many cases such reliance is rewarded, particularly in the case of many cancers, in other cases the results are merely palliative, with short-term outcomes.

Prevention remains something few patients are willing to take on, or doctors and nurses to suggest. There remains an acute-intervention focus in the system and by most practitioners, given that the majority are educated and work in acute facilities. Prevention often demands altered lifestyles, including diet, exercise and changes to work and relaxation patterns, somehow more difficult to manage than taking a pill or undergoing the knife. Doctors cannot write a prescription for it.

A current example of a preventive approach to a significant clinical problem which is changing attitudes and overturning entrenched clinical behaviours is that of pain management. A recent National Health and Medical Research Council (NH&MRC) report *Acute pain management: information for general practitioners* noted the cost of severe unrelieved pain to be more than $10 billion a year, leading to chronic pain if not treated appropriately in the first instance.[12] While research for some time had produced evidence that over 50 per cent of pain remains unrelieved after surgery, post-natally, in the young and the old, it is obvious that we had not addressed this major clinical problem through appropriate preventive management.

Interestingly, evidence pointed to outdated assumptions of practitioners as the main cause of unrelieved pain. These assumptions included beliefs such as 'severe pain is something to be endured as an inevitable consequence of an illness, injury or operation' or 'pain killers make it harder to diagnose an illness' or 'some are worried about side effects or possible addiction'.[13] As Professor Michael Cousins, Head of the Pain Management and Research Centre, Royal North Shore Hospital and the University of Sydney, states, 'No-one should have to live with severe debilitating pain. If someone is suffering, pain relief should be a basic human right.'[14] This is but one example of the way in which practices can have a limited basis in scientific evidence and are resistant to change.

While there is no doubt that individual change is essential if a culture is to change, there also needs to be a system-wide approach to changing professional practice. As Jenny Thomas, assistant secretary to the National Health Priorities and Quality Branch, points out:

> Our medical education system (and I would add our nursing education system) and our model of healthcare provision emphasise the responsibility of the individual clinicians for the care they give and its outcomes for individual patients: and underemphasise the contribution made to quality of care by the system of care. The downside of this is that blame and the willingness to bear it often falls on individual clinicians. They feel, and we expect, that they should have all the answers.[15]

This climate of blame has always existed to the detriment of the system of care and patient outcomes. The fact that the need to blame individuals is still entrenched, as evidenced in recent NSW Health Care Complaints investigations into Canterbury and Dubbo hospitals, highlights the intransigent nature of health care as a system. As Thomas suggests, such a climate leads to a 'paralysis in clinical practice improvement work by clinicians'.[16]

TOWARDS A BETTER SYSTEM

In his analysis of a successful health system, John Wyn Owen[17] outlines the key elements as: continuous planning, implementation and monitoring; investment in education and training of staff; access to up-to-date information technology; recognition of excellence; research-based and outcome-directed practice; and critical evaluation of all aspects of the system. He emphasises the importance of attitudes and practices which patients continually raised in their stories of care.

This is reflected in D's story. Despite the less than ideal context in which she received care for her back injury, her overall experience was a positive one because of the attitude and clinical competence of her doctor:

> Primarily because it [severe back pain and a limp] wasn't getting any better I went to see a neurosurgeon. He was very pleasant but he kept me waiting for 2½ hours, and that was his standard behaviour at every appointment. And we were all people in the same sort of pain and back problems and we sat in his waiting room. And it was interesting because people couldn't sit and you had this collection of people prowling around. There were no couches—there were scooped-back chairs, and you couldn't sit back in these chairs, you were sitting on the edge of the chairs and then prowling around. And it's the sort of arrogance that really makes me angry actually. 'I'm much more important than you are', which I find really irritating.

Yet, as she continues:

> When I did get to see him he was very personable and was very thorough and he gave me a lot of confidence because the idea of having back surgery was just terrifying. I didn't want to do it. I think it was to do with the level of explanation he gave. He knew where he was, he knew what he was talking about, he was really able to explain the procedure. He showed me visually what the procedure was going to be, where he was going to enter the spinal cord, what he was going to remove. We talked through all that. He talked about potential adverse events, he laid out potential side effects . . . he talked about the value of trying alternative care and he left the decision making to me.

The confidence D felt after such a skilled medical consultancy made up for the frustration she felt while waiting for such a long period of time. As she told me, 'I realised that once you got in to see him, he gave you his total attention. And that is why we waited so long.'

D went on to have quite successful surgery, although her time in hospital was very difficult, with poor quality nursing care and subsequently poor pain relief and gross discomfort. She required further admissions due to complications which she had been warned about and accepted as the risk one takes when undergoing such major surgery. These health outcomes were totally acceptable to her, but incompetent and insensitive staff were not.

What D's story highlights is how important it is for patients to feel included and respected by those who care for them. And this principle is not one applicable only at the level of specific individual care, but is one that needs to be extrapolated to the community as a whole. In delivering the 1999 Sydney Sax Oration, Chris Sidoti, lawyer and human rights advocate, stated that: 'Healthy communities are created when people of all generations are included within that community, without discrimination and with generosity, tolerance and respect.'[18] Sidoti states what I and many of my colleagues in health care believe, but this goal requires more than just goodwill on the part of individuals within the system to achieve.

CONCLUSION

'You know we doctors think we know it all—but we don't even begin to understand the mystery of disease and death. When individuals are ready to die they decide the date and the time.' Professor N spoke quietly to me and one of my daughters as we contemplated the difficult questions surrounding death when someone is also having an opiate such as morphine for pain relief. Was my mother's death the result of the morphine or was it the disease process? This conversation was reminiscent of many I'd had with relatives; but this time I was on their side of the question.

Sue's story began this book and her story is a continuing one of uncertainty in the joy of her new life. It is fitting therefore that the book ends with the uncertainty of professional practice so poignantly expressed by an expert not only in medicine but also in the uncertainty of life and death. Increasingly, patients and practitioners are aware of, and must come to terms with, the uncertainty which surrounds illness and disease. It is a daily companion which we fight and even cover up in order to retain control over what is now an increasingly risky business—the business of health.

Between 1960 and the year 2000, society was certainly transformed—technological innovation and the commodification of public institutions being two areas which have had major impacts on the cost and funding of health care. More educated professionals and patients, along with the changing place of women in society, have also altered the way the system is socially and politically constructed. Today disillusionment with the system is as much a part of professional practice as it is of patient critique.

Take M, a registered nurse working in an isolated community for many years and trying to make a difference with little support and even overt opposition. She sighed as she began her story:

I'm just disillusioned with the whole process. Recently I was looking after an Aboriginal girl. She came in with her mother. She was only 12 years of age and had been abducted and raped over many days. She was pregnant, had Hepatitis B and C and wanted a termination. The Department of Community Services (DOCS) rang me and asked me to help her because their role is protective so they could not deal with a termination. I then had to find a doctor who would do the termination, contact Forensic Pathology because we needed evidence for the trial as they had caught the guy who did it, and organise transport for the mother, auntie and the girl to the nearest town. I had to get the blood tests because the local general practitioners are both men and the girl and her mum wouldn't go to them.

As I listened to M's story of her work as a nurse in a rural town, the discrepancies within the health care system and the inequities in our society were once more illuminated.

If you're not willing to undertake what really isn't your designated role as a community nurse, then this young girl would have continued on with her pregnancy or had a backyard abortion. I gave her counselling—I couldn't get an Aboriginal nurse—but later I got an Aboriginal midwife who was great. I had to organise accommodation and transport back on a Saturday and the Department of Community Services (DOCS) weren't going to pay for it. I said, 'Excuse me! You have Emergency funding—I have no funding.' They claimed that they were into protection and couldn't fund an abortion.

While initially employed as a Community Nurse on an annual salary of $30 000, M now also works as the Early Discharge nurse for the small local hospital, is the Early Childhood Nurse for the community, and has become the de facto Aboriginal health nurse because the Aboriginal population trust her. As she told me: 'Even the GPs ask me where to refer Aboriginal patients.' She works in

an old bedroom in the hospital with no proper lighting, no telephone or computer. This is where she sees her clients. Despite
travelling around the community, she isn't provided with facilities
such as a mobile phone unless she shares one with the mental
health team. For M, the future means even more responsibility
without any increase in resources:

> This year DOCS will be handing over more responsibility to
> nurses, doctors and teachers. With no social worker I do all that
> work as well. I also do guardianship work and we have no Aged
> Care worker. We've just had a case of elder abuse and I had to
> get her out of her home.
>
> That's the trouble with geographical isolation. It's all very
> well to rationalise and regionalise things. When they take the
> workers out of the town problems still happen and someone
> has to deal with it. I can be walking past the maternity unit
> and the maternity buzzer goes off and in I go to help with
> the delivery—and I can be on call because they haven't got
> another midwife—and I also do escorts because they haven't
> got anyone else to go in the ambulance.

M's story is one of many practitioners' stories, both nurses
and doctors, in our isolated communities. Dedicated and competent, they are increasingly frustrated with the lack of access
to expertise and other resources. While those working in large
teaching hospitals feel equally frustrated and have valid reasons
for feeling so, it is usually for very different reasons—such as
not being consulted or having limited access to facilities. For
those in isolated communities it is about having no one to
consult and no facilities such as a telephone. In turn, inequities
for practitioners affect the individuals and communities they care
for daily, either through inadequate facilities or staff who walk
away from the job. Paying attention to those in our system who
are central to communities and hospitals is increasingly important
if we are to retain quality staff to improve the health of communities. Both are essential.

So, is the experience of being sick any different today than it
was in the 1960s? There is little doubt that there have been major
changes within the health care system, mainly brought about by

new technology and the possibilities this has opened for the diagnosis and management of disease. In theory more lives should be saved or extended, complicated surgery should be safer and diagnosis more accurate. It could therefore be assumed that the experience of being ill would now be less traumatic. But there is no clear evidence that this is so. Illness remains a very uncertain and human experience, as many of the stories in this book attest.

Of course, the way in which individuals access the system has also changed. In the 1960s it was still possible to have the local doctor call at home at any time. Today this is rare, particularly at night. Many people do not have a regular general practitioner but instead they visit a hospital emergency department or a private medical centre. This means a loss of continuity in terms of patients' histories over time, making diagnosis at times of acute illness more difficult. Compounding this has been the burgeoning of specialties and specialists which fragments care at the same time as it may improve the management of specific diseases or disorders.

We now live with a system which is full of contradictions. The first is while medical science is perceived as the sole reason for the improving health of our nation in fact it has been demonstrated that the reduction of deaths from infectious diseases such as tuberculosis and whooping cough is directly linked to factors such as adequate housing, clean water, nutrition and smaller families.[1] And this remains so today. Where there is poverty, social and environmental factors are strong determinants of poor health and high mortality rates. Yet we do little about linking these factors either politically or in practice. At the other end of the spectrum, prolonging life through organ donation leaves individuals with the possibility of rejection or other disease because of their drug regime, despite the miracle of a new life. The cost of sophisticated technology and specialisation has driven costs and demand to the point where we are questioning the financial viability of a public system at the same time as a significant number in our community have limited access to even basic health care.

Technology has created the industry of 'anticipatory' medicine which Petr Skrabanek defines as that form of medicine which 'indulges in probablistic speculations about the future risk of so called multifactorial disorders in individuals'.[2] An example of this is contained in the official preventive care guidelines put out by the American College of Physicians for women between 20 and 70 years of age.[3] For an individual this would mean 278 examinations, tests and counselling sessions and this is recommended for a *healthy* woman. The promise of such an approach is that individuals gain control over their lives as long as they modify them according to a set of guidelines. In truth, however, we now divide a person up between specialists for scrutiny with the patient left feeling fragmented and uncertain—far from being in control.

Some things today are certainly for the better. In the main they relate to the way in which individuals are treated and managed. This extends to the way in which a hospital or service is organised and interacts with patients. Recently the experience of being with my eldest daughter during her labour was in direct contrast to my own much more restricted and medicalised births. And even more recently, when the results of my mother's many scans came back, the doctor squatted beside her bed and told us both that she had secondary cancer in her liver. He talked to her about the alternatives for pain relief and left it to her to make the final decision.

During this time I reflected back thirty years to a time when one of my daughters was admitted to a large teaching hospital as a 16-month-old. Frightened and ill, she was isolated in a single room unable to mix with or even see the other children. Visiting was limited to 2 hours a day. Doctors were shadowy figures who could only be accessed through an appointment. As a mother I felt alienated, frightened and anonymous. That experience remains with me as one in which I wondered whether anyone cared— about my daughter or about me.

As I washed my mother and shared her last hours, talking through her life, the contrast was stark. Much had changed in the system and for the better. I felt supported, listened to and understood and she felt cared for and involved in her treatment and her death.

There have also been changes since 1960 which necessitate an increased accountability within the system. This includes the emphasis on consumer involvement, professional accountability for effective outcomes, and scientific evidence rather than myth or traditions as a basis for practices. Such imperatives have forced an awareness of the need to change if we are to survive the increasing demands from all sectors of society, including the political agenda of economic restraint and abdication of social responsibility.

In some arenas over the last few years, there are also signs of a readiness or willingness to negotiate on the more difficult issues of disciplinary territories as it is becoming increasingly clear that alone we cannot begin to meet the needs of patients today, whether that be in a small isolated community, a general practice or a large city teaching hospital. Patients' needs are increasingly complicated due to any one of a multiplicity of reasons, including early discharge, frailer conditions, sophisticated treatments or drug regimes, need for pain relief or ongoing education and rehabilitation. Such coordination of care requires one person in a team who can manage the care across disciplines, contexts and stages of the disease or illness. While this may be the general practitioner it could also be a nurse who is a Case Manager or a Nurse Practitioner. But whoever it is, they also need the support and infrastructure of the team itself. Indeed, we have only just begun to imagine the various models of care available to us if we truly want to provide care which meets the needs of individuals in various contexts and with diverse health concerns. This may be the most exciting challenge for us all in health care today.

In 1960 uncertainty was not an obvious part of the culture— today it is central to much of what passes for health care. And I see this as a positive shift if it forces us to think and act differently, questioning the 'taken for granted' and the ritualistic in the health care culture, seeking evidence and listening to patients who are so often the experts, while acknowledging our own frailties and limitations as experts. Just as we are shifting responsibility to individuals and communities to fund and manage their own health care needs, those of us involved in the health care professions need to take responsibility for our part in this changing culture— a culture which has, in many ways, been able to ignore the impact of social change up until the last decade. But this is no longer possible. Such an entrenched culture has become a major liability in terms of delivering effective health care to those in need. Within and without the system of health care the world has changed dramatically and forever. There is no turning back the clock on technology and the drug cartels, miracle interventions, social change, well-informed patients and well-educated staff. Instead, we need to harness these changes as best we can to meet our ends as providers of high quality care to contemporary communities.

We know that the power to ensure truly healthy communities is best garnered when all interested parties are engaged from the very beginning of the struggle. If we are going to change the unchangeable in the Australian health care system we need a critical mass from all walks of life, rather than fragmented groups with vested interests, which is a feature of our Australian landscape.

The question to be answered is a collective one: what values and models do we want sustained and reflected in the system we call health care? This question constitutes the core of this book, a book which was never intended to be a comprehensive text on the health care system, but rather one which reflects a range of personal experiences: my own, those of my colleagues and, above all, those of the patients we have cared for. It is, after all, the patients who must ultimately judge whether we care.

ENDNOTES

INTRODUCTION

1 J. Kirner & M. Rayner, *The Women's Power Handbook*, Viking Press, Melbourne, 1999.
2 M. Florez, 'Home is where the heart and business is', *Sunday Telegraph*, 5 March 2000, p. 7.
3 Kirner & Rayner, p. 22. (For a thorough analysis of changes for women in terms of employment, financial status and representation see Kirner & Rayner, *The Women's Power Handbook*, Viking Press, Melbourne, 1999.)
4 W.E. May, *The Patient's Ordeal*, Indiana University Press, Bloomington, 1994, p. 21.
5 R.H. Tawney cited in D. Dutton, *Worse than the Disease: Pitfalls of Medical Progress*, reprint Cambridge University Press, New York, 1992, p. 10.

CHAPTER 1—THE PATIENT AS INFORMED CONSUMER

1 P. Phelan, 'Promoting quality and efficiency in health services', Guest Editorial, *Better Health Outcomes*, vol. 5, no. 4, Summer 1999, pp. 1–2.
2 Editorial, *Health and Development*, no. 181, August 1998, p. 2.
3 'Enough to make you sick: How income and environment

affect health', *National Health Strategy Research Paper No. 1*, Treble Press, ACT, September 1992.

4   'NSW Health: The year in review 1997/98', Annual Report, NSW Health, NSW Health Department, Sydney, 1998, p. 7.

5   R. Moynihan, *Too Much Medicine: The Business of Health and its Risks for You*, ABC Books, Sydney, 1998.

6   B. Hall, 'A matter of life and death out in Sydney's west', *Sydney Morning Herald*, 8 January 1999, p. 13.

7   A. Phelan, 'Culture, cure: orthodoxy embraces alternative medicine. Health for Life 1', *Sydney Morning Herald*, 21 October 1997, pp. H1–4.

8   Phelan, p. H1.

9   S. Okie, 'Alternative treatments turning people around', *Sydney Morning Herald*, 12 November 1998.

10 C. Johnston, 'Doctors in distress', *Sunday Life*, *Sun-Herald*, 8 November 1998, pp. 10–11.

11 M. Walton, 'Anatomy of a complaint—error of judgment or professional misconduct?', *Health Investigator*, 1:3, February 1998, p. 1.

12 Walton, p. 1.

CHAPTER 2—THE CHANGING STATUS OF WOMEN

1   E. Showalter, 'Florence Nightingale's feminist complaint: Women, religion and suggestions for thought', *Signs*, vol. 6, pp. 395–412.

2   H. Wilkinson & M. Howard, *Tomorrow's Women*, Demos, London, 1997.

3   R. Pringle, 'Family, kith, and kin' in B. Caine (ed.), *Australian Feminism: A Companion*, Oxford University Press, Melbourne, 1998, p. 98.

4   Wilkinson & Howard, p. 9.

5   D. Mitchell, 'Wages and employment', *Tomorrow's Women*, Demos, London, 1997, p. 362.

6   R. Birrell cited in S. Loane & A. Horin, 'Women take the clever path to the top. Australian women: The vital statistics', *Sydney Morning Herald*, 20 April 1998, p. 1.

7   Kelly cited in B. Arndt, 'Degrees of strain', *Sydney Morning Herald*, 13 October 1997, p. 15.

8   Mitchell, pp. 363–4.

9   P. Staunton, *Budget Estimates and Related Papers*, NSW State Government, 18 October 1995.

10 M.P. Donahue, *Nursing, The Finest Art: An Illustrated History*, C V Mosby, St Louis, 1985, p. 63.

11 J. Barnett Wilson, 'Project 2000: Australian regrading', *Nursing Times*, 28 September 1998, p. 39.

12 L. Brereton, Media release issued from the Office of the Minister for Health, November 1983.

13 A. Summers, 'Twin drives for twin needs', *Australian Nurses Journal*, 14:10, May 1985, p. 37.

14 Y.B. Lim, 'Difference between doctors and nurses', *Sydney Morning Herald*, 24 September 1997.

15 J. Lumby & J. Zetlar, 'Image: Symbolism in nursing', paper presented at The NSW College of Nursing Oration Conference, Nursing's Image—Yesterday, Today & Tomorrow, September 1989.

16 NSW Health Department *Issues Paper* relating to specialty nursing vacancies. Study undertaken by KPMG Peat Marwick, 1995.

17 D. Picone, J. Lumby & J. Lawler, 'Improving patients' outcomes project', *Draft Final Report NSW Nurses Registration Board*, December 1998.

18 K. Walker, 'Harassment, staff relationships and personnel development in NSW healthcare', NSW College of Nursing Report, October 1997 (unpublished).

19 M.C. Lovell, 'Silent but perfect "partners": medicine's use and abuse of women', *Advances in Nursing Science*, vol. 3, no. 2, p. 29.

20 R. Pringle, *Sex and Medicine*, Cambridge University Press, Melbourne, 1998.

CHAPTER 3—THE IMPACT OF TECHNOLOGY

1   E. Tenner, *Why Things Bite Back: New Technology and the Revenge Effect*, Fourth Estate, London, 1996.

2 D.W. Bates, 'Frequency, consequences and prevention of adverse drug events', *Journal of Quality in Clinical Practice*, vol. 19, no. 1, 1999, pp. 13–17.

3 E.E. Roughhead, 'The nature and extent of drug related hospitalisations in Australia', *Journal of Quality in Clinical Practice*, vol. 19, no. 1, 1999, pp. 19–22.

4 R. Moynihan, *Too Much Medicine? The Business of Health and its Risks for You*, ABC Books, Sydney, 1998, p. 35.

5 NSW Innovation Council, 'Biotechnology in NSW: Opportunities and challenges', report to the NSW government, NSW Department of State and Regional Development, 1998.

6 S. Crowe, 'A nation of drug takers', *University of Sydney News*, vol. 31, no. 8, 1999, p. 1.

7 J. Lumby, 'Liver transplantation: The death/life paradox', *International Journal of Nursing Practice*, vol. 3, no. 4, December 1997, pp. 231–8.

8 *Better Health Outcomes Newsletter*, Health Services Quality and Outcomes Branch, vol. 4, no. 4, 4 December 1998.

CHAPTER 4—THE COMMODIFICATION OF
HEALTH CARE

1 J. Whelan, 'Hospital unable to cope as it bleeds from fiscal cuts', *Sydney Morning Herald*, 13 July 1999, p. 6.

2 J. Whelan, 'Sydney's sickest hospital', *Sydney Morning Herald*, 9 July 1999, p. 1.

3 J. Baird & A. Bernoth, 'Hospital emergency', *Sydney Morning Herald*, 12 July 1999, p. 1.

4 S. Sax, *A Strife of Interests: Politics and Policies in Australian Health Services*, Allen & Unwin, Sydney, 1984.

5 G.R. Palmer & S.D. Short, *Health Care Public Policy: An Australian Analysis*, Macmillan, Melbourne, 1989, p. 54.

6 Sax.

7 A. Crichton citing T. Fox, *Slowly Taking Control: Australian governments and health care provision 1788–1988*, Allen & Unwin, Sydney, 1990, p. 44.

8 Crichton, p. 85.

9   J. Dewdney, 'Health services in Australia' in M.W. Raffel (ed.), *Comparative Health Systems: Descriptive Analyses of Fourteen National Health Systems*, Pennsylvania University Press, Pennsylvania, 1984, pp. 1–54.

10 Crichton.

11 Sax, p. 55.

12 Sax, p. 29.

13 NSW Health, 'A review of health', *Independent Pricing and Regulatory Tribunal of NSW*, QVB Post Office, Sydney, November 1998.

14 NSW Health.

15 NSW Health, p. 4.

16 Newsletter, 'Time for a national rethink of Australia's healthcare system', Australian Healthcare Association, 16 July 1999.

17 'Time for a national rethink . . .', p. 12.

18 S. Schwartz, 'Health care system books in for reality check', *Australian*, 27 April 1999, p. 32.

19 J. Robotham, 'Caesarian births rise to one in five', *Sydney Morning Herald*, 31 March 1999, p. 2.

20 Crichton, p. 86.

21 K. Suter, 'Social capital', paper given at Real Reform or Political Rhetoric, The Health Services Association's annual conference, 9 July 1999.

22 J. Hyde, 'Responses to globalisation—Rethinking equity and health', paper given at Real Reform or Political Rhetoric, The Health Services Association's Annual Conference, 9 July 1999.

23 Hyde.

24 J. Lomas, 'Social capital and health: Implications for public health and epidemiology', *Social Science Medicine*, vol. 478, no. 9, 1998, pp. 1181–8; J.A. Dixon, 'National R&D collaboration on health and socioeconomic status for Australia', *First Discussion Paper*, National Centre for Epidemiology and Population Health, January 1999; J. Raulston Saul, *The Unconscious Civilisation*, Penguin Books, Melbourne, 1997, p. 14.

25 G.R. Palmer & S.D. Short, *Health Care and Public Policy. An Australian Analysis*, Macmillan, Hong Kong, 1989.

26 S. Leeder, 'Dark side to the future of Medicare', *Sydney Morning Herald*, 23 July 1999, p. 15.

27 F. Brenchley, 'Picture of health', *Bulletin*, 8 June 1999, pp. 24–6.

28 G. Anders, *Health Against Wealth: HMOs and the Breakdown of Medical Trust*, Houghton Mifflin Co., New York, 1996.

29 J. Braithwaite & J.I. Westbrook, 'For richer, for poorer, in sickness and in health: International issues of quality and cost', *Australian Hospital Association Management Issues*, July 1992, ISSN 1038–4995.

CHAPTER 5—THE PROBLEM OF EQUITY AND ACCESS

1 Quality Framework, NSW Department of Health, 1999, p. 23.

2 AIHW, *Australia's Health 1998*, 6th biennial health report of the Australian Institute of Health and Welfare', *Australian Institute of Health and Welfare*, Cat. no. AUS 10, Canberra, p. 205.

3 AIHW, p. 139.

4 S. Leeder, *Healthy Medicine: Challenges Facing Australia's Health Services*, Allen & Unwin, Sydney, 1999, p. 3.

5 H. Pampling & G. Gregory, *Leaping the Boundary Fence*, Proceedings, 5th National Rural Health Conference, National Rural Health Alliance, 14–17 March, Adelaide, 1999, p. 148.

6 Leeder, p. 5.

7 Pampling & Gregory, p. 101.

8 Pampling & Gregory, p. 130.

9 AIHW, p. 40.

10 *Australian Social Trends 1999*, Australian Bureau of Statistics, Cat. no. 4102.0, Canberra, p. 11.

11 *Talking Better Health With People from Non-English Speaking Backgrounds*, Centre for Development and Innovation in Health (CDIH); Commonwealth of Australia, Victoria, 1998, p. 6.

12 'Removing cultural and language barriers to health', *National Health Strategy Issues Paper No. 6*, March 1993, p. 9.

13   'Removing cultural and language barriers to health', p. 10.
14   Leeder, p. 23.
15   AIHW, *Health Expenditure Bulletin*, No. 15, Australia's health services expenditure to 1997–98, Canberra (Health and Welfare Expenditure Series), ISSN 1329–2137, 1999.
16   F. Baum, 'Social capital and health: Implications for health in rural Australia', *Leaping the Boundary Fence*, 5th National Rural Health Conference, National Rural Health Alliance, 14–17 March, Adelaide, 1999, p. 103.

CHAPTER 6—DESIGNING HEALTH CARE

1   J. Deeble, 'Learning from the Chinook', *In Touch*, Newsletter of the Public Health Association of Australia Inc., Curtin, ACT, December 1999, pp. 6–7.
2   AIHW, *Australia's Health 1998*, 6th biennial health report of the Australian Institute of Health and Welfare, Cat. no. AUS 10, Commonwealth of Australia, Canberra, 1998, p. 175.
3   T.V. Lieshout, 'The destruction of our public hospitals', *New Doctor*, Winter, 1998, p. 18.
4   M. Metherell, 'Doctors should declare fees up front, says AVCC', *Sydney Morning Herald*, 13 April 2000, p. 5.
5   J. Kerin, 'Doctors slash costs as no-gap claims surge', *Australian*, 9 December 1999, p. 5.
6   J. Hewson, 'Taxing health of reform process', *Australian Financial Review*, 25 May 1998, p. 16.
7   AIHW.
8   M. Wilkinson, 'Bitter pill', *Sydney Morning Herald: News Review*, 4 December 1999, p. 42.
9   AIHW, p. 29.
10   AIHW, p. 17.
11   M. Metherell, 'Health link to income on the rise', *Sydney Morning Herald*, 15 April 2000, p. 7.
12   'Enough to make you sick: How income and environment affect health', *National Health Strategy Research Paper No. 1*, Treble Press, ACT, ISSN 1038–9229, September 1992, p. 10.
13   A. Horin, 'Australians turn the other cheek to poverty', *Sydney Morning Herald*, 24 December 1999, p. 23.

14 M. Metherell, 'Rural doctors call: Raise our Medicare fee', *Sydney Morning Herald*, 5 February 1999, p. 11.

15 J. Wyn Owen, 'Introduction' in M. Warner, *Redesigning Health Services: Reducing the Zone of Delusion*, The Nuffield Trust, Series No. 1, Nuffield Trust, London, 1997, p. 6.

Chapter 7—Major challenges

1 J. Deeble, 'Learning from the Chinook', *In Touch*, Newsletter of the Public Health Association of Australia Inc., PHAA, Curtin, ACT, December 1999, pp. 6–7.

2 Commonwealth of Australia, *Rethinking Nursing: National Nursing Workforce Forum*, Commonwealth Department of Health and Aged Care, Canberra, ISBN 0642415803, 2000.

3 G. Anders, *Health Against Wealth: HMOs and the Breakdown of Medical Trust*, Houghton Mifflin Co., New York, 1996.

4 'USA: Marketplace economics transforming US hospitals and driving local collaboration. Systemic change drives health care associations back to the drawing board', *Healthcover: For Decision Makers in Health*, Healthdata Services, vol. 8, no. 1, February–March 1998, p. 37.

5 M. Wooldridge, 'Another round of measures to shore up the private sector', *Healthcover: For Decision Makers in Health*, vol. 8, no. 1, February–March 1998, p. 11.

6 Wooldridge, p. 11.

7 D. Hindle & J. Braithwaite, 'Blair's Labour and Howard's Coalition: On the same path to health?', *Healthcover: For Decision Makers in Health*, vol. 8, no. 1, February–March 1998, p. 15.

8 J. Kerin, 'Record 8m with health coverage', *Australian*, 15 August 2000, p. 3.

9 J. Millar, 'The federal government tax package', *Health Forum*, no. 45, September 1998, p. 17.

10 K. Davidson, 'The long march to private health', Opinion, *Age*, 28 September 2000, p. 11.

11 Hindle & Braithwaite, p. 17.

12 G. Jacobsen, 'Amanda's silent world: A profile of a system not coping', *Sydney Morning Herald*, 27 November 1999, p. 6.

13 C. Donaldson, 'Why a National Health Service? The economic rationale', *Institute of Public Policy Research*, Emphasis, London, 1998, p. 7.
14 Donaldson, p. 7.
15 Donaldson.
16 WHO, 'WHO primary healthcare systems and services for the 21st century', Statement of the Seventh Consultative Committee on Organisation of Health Systems Based on Primary Health Care, Geneva, 1997.
17 Millar, p. 17.
18 C. Krestensen, 'Privately funded health care—What's it really costing us?', *Health Forum*, no. 45, September 1998, p. 119.
19 See S. Sax, *A Strife of Interests: Politics and Policies in Australian Health Services*, Allen & Unwin, Sydney, 1984, for a comprehensive discussion.

CHAPTER 8—FUTURE DELIVERY OF CARE

1 C. Sidoti, 'Rights for all: Building inclusive communities for all generations', Public Health Association of Australia Sax Oration delivered by Chris Sidoti, 18 November 1999, published in *In Touch*, Newsletter of the Public Health Association of Australia Inc., vol. 16, no. 1, December 1999, p. 2.
2 M. Walton 'Why Australia's doctors need a regular check-up', *Sydney Morning Herald*, 17 January 2000.
3 Walton, p. 3.
4 Walton, p. 4.
5 J. Israel & J. Vaughan, 'Nursing homes rated "unacceptable"', *Sydney Morning Herald*, 2 March 2000, p. 4.
6 M. Leeder, 'All for one and one for all? The ethics of resource allocation for health care', Point of View, *Australian Medical Journal*, vol. 147, 20 July 1987, p. 69.
7 F. Baum, 'Social capital and health: Implications for health in Rural Australia', paper published in conference proceedings, *5th National Rural Health Conference*, 1999.
8 J. Menadue, Chairman's Message in *Report of the NSW Health Council: A Better Health System for NSW, 03/2000*, Better

Health Centre, Gladesville, NSW, February 2000, p. iv.

9   A. Wilson, 'Message from the Chair', *National Public Health Partnership News*, Issue 10, Melbourne, December 1999.

10 S. Sax, *A Strife of Interests: Politics and Policies in Australian Health Services*, Allen & Unwin, Sydney, 1984.

11 M. Ragg, 'Healthier hearts remain mystery', *Sydney Morning Herald*, 26 February 1999, p. 11.

12 NH&MRC, 'GPs in front line for effective acute pain relief', *NHMRC News: A Biannual Commentary on Australian Healthcare Issues*, Issue 3, vol. 1, September 1999, p. 1.

13 NH&MRC, p. 2.

14 NH&MRC, p. 2.

15 J. Thomas, 'Quality and safety: A "beyond blame" focus', Keynote Address to the Australian Association for Quality in Health Care conference, Adelaide, June 15 1999, in *Better Health Outcomes. National Health Priorities and Quality Branch*, Commonwealth Department of Health and Aged Care, vol. 5, Summer 1999, p. 4.

16 Thomas, p. 4.

17 J. Wyn Owen in M. Warner, *Redesigning Health Services: Reducing the Zone of Delusion*, The Nuffield Series No. 1, Nuffield Trust, London, 1997.

18 Sidoti, p. 5.

CONCLUSION

1   P. Skrabanek citing T. McKeown in *The Death of Humane Medicine and the Rise of Coercive Healthism*, Social Affairs Unit, St Edmundsbury Press, Suffolk, 1994, p. 21.

2   Skrabanek, p. 32.

3   Skrabanek, p. 33.

INDEX

Aboriginal and Torres Strait
    Islander health
    inequities, 68–9, 76–7
    initiatives, 91
ageing population, 93
    care of, 92–3
    funding of, 93
    Home and Community
        Care (HACC), 92
'alternative' health care, 12–14
    contemporary move to,
        12–15
    incorporation within
        nursing and medicine,
        14–15
Area Health Services, 101
Australian health care system,
    7–12
Australian Medical Association
    (AMA), 57–8, 60, 115

Baum, Fran, 87
British Medical Association
    (BMA), 57, 59

Canadian health care system,
    90, 110–11

commodification of health
    care, 54–71
    impact on delivery of care,
        60–3
    impact on patients, 63–4
    politics of, 56–60
consumer information, 1–8
consumer movement, 10–11
    Consumer Focus
        Collaboration, 4
Cormack, Mark, 64–5
cost-shifting, 92, 96
Cousins, Professor Michael,
    135

doctor–patient relationship,
    15–18
Duckett, Professor Steven,
    118

Enhanced Primary Care
    Package (EPCP), 132
equity of access, 72–88
    discriminatory practices,
        75–7, 82
    distribution of services,
        85–8

isolated communities, 77–81
patients with disabilities,
81–5
socio-economically
disadvantaged, 126
United Nations Human
Development Index,
95–6
evidence-based medicine, 8

funding
alternative models, 110–11
cost versus quality, 60–71
distribution of, 95–6,
127–33
federal/state, 91
inequity of, 121–5
Lifetime Health Cover, 118
managed care, 115–16
politics of, 56–60
public/private, 90, 118–19
future of health care, 126–37

general practitioners, 99

health care
cost of, 69–71
definitions, 8–9
illness model, 8–9, 11–12,
94–5
primary health model, 10
health care complaints, 6, 17
mechanisms for, 6
NSW Health Care
Complaints
Commission, 6

Independent Pricing and
Regulatory Tribunal, 60

international models of care,
110–24

Lawrence, Professor Jim,
xvi–xvii
Leeder, Professor Stephen, 68,
76, 129–30
Little, Professor Miles, 17–18

Medicare, 91–2
Menadue, John, 132
models of care, 96–107
case management, 111–13
community, 101
early discharge, 101, 106
hospital in the home, 101
impact on patients, 102–7
multidisciplinary, 98–9
Nurse Practitioner, 100–1
practitioner driven, 97
primary care, 99–100
primary health, 99–100, 106
specialist, 102–3
task centred, 97
women's health, 98, 105

National Aboriginal Health
Strategy, 76
National Expert Advisory
Group on Safety and
Quality in Australian
Health Care, 52
National Health Strategy
(1992), 9, 95
National Public Health
Partnership, 133
NSW Department of
Health Quality
Framework, 73

NSW Health Council report, 132
Nurse Practitioner
  backlash, 28, 31–2
  legislation, 26, 100–1
  NSW Independent Nurse Practitioner role, 113–15
nurses
  Case Managers, 31, 111–13
  changing role of, 41–3
  Clinical Nurse Consultants, 32, 41
  education of, 26–8
  past practices of, 1
  shortage of, 29, 61
  traditional view of, 1–2, 29

Owen, John Wyn, 107, 135

patients
  as informed consumers, 1–18
  attitudes to practitioners, 3–8
  past attitudes to, 2, 3
  perceptions of health, 8–15
  relationship to doctors, 15–18
  rights, 1
Pharmaceutical Benefits Act (1947), 58
Pharmaceutical Benefits Advisory Committee (PBAC), 93
Pharmaceutical Benefits Scheme, 93
pharmacology, errors, 44

primary health care, lack of funding, 2
Pringle, Rosemary, 20, 34–5

Ralston Saul, John, 65
remote area health
  access to care, 85
  doctor shortages in, 78
  inequities compared with urban care, 77–81, 85
  primary health, nursing in, 10, 78, 81, 101, 105, 106
Residential Aged Care Act (1997), 128
resource distribution, 94–6

Sax, Sydney, 56
Sidoti, Chris, 126
Staunton, Patricia, 24
Suter, Dr Keith, 66

technology, 36–53
  and litigation, 45
  cost of high-tech health care, 44–8
  ethics of, 48
  history of developments, 38–41
  impact on patient care and patients, 41–9, 51–2

UK health care system, 117
US health care system, 44–5, 115
user pays, 92

Walton, Merilyn, 17
Wilson, Dr Andrew, 133

women
  and health, 19–35
  and medical intervention, 33, 65
  and nursing, 24–9
  changing status of, 20–3
  health centres, 98

impact of change for patients, 30–5
Sex Discrimination Act (1975), 21
Women's Electoral Lobby, 21
women's movement, 20–1